The Hand, Its Mechanism and Vital Endowments As Evincing Design

Charles Bell

THE BRIDGEWATER TREATISES

ON THE POWER, WISDOM, AND GOODNESS OF GOD
AS MANIFESTED IN THE CREATION.

TREATISE IV.

THE HAND, ITS MECHANISM AND VITAL ENDOWMENTS,

AS EVINCING DESIGN.

BY SIR CHARLES BELL, K. G. H. F. R. S. L. & E.

THE HAND,

ITS MECHANISM AND VITAL ENDOWMENTS,

AS EVINCING DESIGN.

BY

SIR CHARLES BELL, K. G. H.

F.R.S. L.&E.

PHILADELPHIA:

CAREY, LEA & BLANCHARD.

1833.

NOTICE.

THE series of Treatises, of which the present is one, is published under the following circumstances :

The RIGHT HONOURABLE and REVEREND FRANCIS HENRY, EARL of BRIDGEWATER, died in the month of February, 1829; and by his last Will and Testament, bearing date the 25th of February, 1825, he directed certain Trustees therein named to invest in the public funds the sum of Eight thousand pounds sterling : this sum, with the accruing dividends thereon, to be held at the disposal of the President, for the time being, of the Royal Society of London, to be paid to the person or persons nominated by him. The Testator further directed, that the person or persons selected by the said President should be appointed to write, print, and publish one thousand copies of a work *On the Power, Wisdom, and Goodness of God, as manifested in the Creation ; illustrating such work by all reasonable arguments, as for instance the variety and formation of God's creatures in the animal, vegetable, and mineral kingdoms ; the effect of digestion, and thereby of conversion ; the construction of the hand of man, and an infinite variety of other arguments ; as also by discoveries ancient and modern, in arts, sciences, and the whole extent of literature.* He desired, moreover, that the profits arising from the sale of the works so published should be paid to the authors of the works.

The late President of the Royal Society, Davies Gilbert, Esq. requested the assistance of his Grace the Archbishop of Canterbury and of the Bishop of London, in determining upon the best mode of carrying into effect the intentions of the Testator. Acting with their advice, and with the concurrence of a nobleman immediately connected with the deceased, Mr. Davies Gilbert appointed the following eight gentlemen to write separate Treatises on the different branches of the subject as here stated :

THE REV. THOMAS CHALMERS, D. D.
PROFESSOR OF DIVINITY IN THE UNIVERSITY OF EDINBURGH.
ON THE ADAPTATION OF EXTERNAL NATURE TO THE MORAL AND INTELLECTUAL CONSTITUTION OF MAN.

JOHN KIDD, M. D. F. R. S.
REGIUS PROFESSOR OF MEDICINE IN THE UNIVERSITY OF OXFORD.
ON THE ADAPTATION OF EXTERNAL NATURE TO THE PHYSICAL CONDITION OF MAN.

THE REV. WILLIAM WHEWELL, M. A. F. R. S.
FELLOW OF TRINITY COLLEGE, CAMBRIDGE.
ON ASTRONOMY AND GENERAL PHYSICS.

SIR CHARLES BELL, K. H. F. R. S.
THE HAND: ITS MECHANISM AND VITAL ENDOWMENTS AS EVINCING DESIGN.

PETER MARK ROGET, M. D.
FELLOW OF AND SECRETARY TO THE ROYAL SOCIETY.
ON ANIMAL AND VEGETABLE PHYSIOLOGY.

THE REV. WILLIAM BUCKLAND, D. D. F. R. S.
CANON OF CHRIST CHURCH, AND PROFESSOR OF GEOLOGY IN THE UNIVERSITY OF OXFORD.
ON GEOLOGY AND MINERALOGY.

THE REV. WILLIAM KIRBY, M. A. F. R. S.
ON THE HISTORY, HABITS, AND INSTINCTS OF ANIMALS.

WILLIAM PROUT, M. D. F. R. S.
ON CHEMISTRY, METEOROLOGY, AND THE FUNCTION OF DIGESTION.

His Royal Highness the Duke of Sussex, President of the Royal Society, having desired that no unnecessary delay should take place in the publication of the above mentioned treatises, they will appear at short intervals, as they are ready for publication.

PREFACE.

WHEN one has to maintain an argument, he will be listened to more willingly if he is known to be unbiassed, and to express his natural sentiments. The reflexions contained in these pages have not been suggested by the occasion of the Bridgewater Treatises, but arose, long ago, in a course of study, directed to other objects. An anatomical teacher, who is himself aware of the higher bearings of his science, can hardly neglect the opportunity which the demonstrations before him afford, of making an impression upon the minds of those young men who, for the most part, receive the elements of their professional education from him; and he is naturally led to indulge in such trains of reflexion, as will be found in this essay.

So far back as the year 1813, the late excellent vicar of Kensington, Mr. Rennell, attended the author's lectures, and found him engaged in maintaining the principles of the English school of Physiology, and in exposing the futility of the opinions of those French philosophers and physiologists, who represented life as the mere physical result of certain combinations and actions of parts, by them termed Organization.

That gentleman thought that the subject admitted of an argument which it became him to use, in his office of " Christian Advocate."* This will show the

* An office in the University of Cambridge.

reader that the sentiments and the views, which a
sense of duty to the young men about him induced
the author to deliver, and which Mr. Rennell heard
only by accident, arose naturally out of those studies.

It was at the desire of the Lord Chancellor that the
author wrote the essay on " Animal Mechanics ;" and
it was probably from a belief that the author felt
the importance of the subjects touched upon in that
essay, that his lordship was led to do him the further honour of asking him to join with him in illustrating the " Natural Theology" of Dr. Paley.

That request was especially important, as showing,
that the conclusions, to which the author had arrived, were not the peculiar or accidental suggestions of
professional feeling, nor of solitary study, which is so
apt to lead to enthusiasm, but that the powerful and
masculine mind of Lord Brougham was directed to
the same object : that he, who in early life was distinguished for his successful prosecution of science,
and who has never forgotten her interests amidst
the most arduous and active duties of his high station,
encouraged and partook of these sentiments.

Thus, from at first maintaining that design and
benevolence were every where visible in the natural
world, circumstances have gradually drawn the author to support these opinions more ostentatiously and
elaborately than was his original wish.

The author cannot conceal from himself the disad-
vantages to which he is exposed in coming before the
public, not only with a work, in some measure extra-
professional, but with associates, distinguished by

classical elegance of style, as well as by science. He must entreat the reader to remember that he was, early and long, devoted to the study of anatomy; and with a feeling (right or wrong) that it surpassed all other studies, in interest and usefulness. This made him negligent of those acquirements which would have better fitted him for the honourable association in which he has been placed: and no one can feel more deeply that the suggestions which occur in the intervals of an active professional life, must always be unfavourably contrasted with what comes of the learned leisure of a College.

The author has to acknowledge his obligation to Davies Gilbert, Esq. late President of the Royal Society, for having assigned to him a task of so much interest. When he undertook it, he thought only of the pleasure of pursuing these investigations, and perhaps too little of what the public were entitled to expect from an Essay composed in circumstances so peculiar, and forming a part in " this great argument."

CONTENTS.

ADDITIONAL ILLUSTRATIONS.

APPENDIX.

THE HAND,

ITS MECHANISM AND VITAL ENDOW-
MENTS, AS EVINCING DESIGN.

CHAPTER I.

IF we contemplate any natural object, especially any part of animated nature, fully and in all its bearings, we can arrive only at this conclusion : that there is design in the mechanical construction, benevolence shown in the living properties, and that good predominates : we shall perceive that the sensibilities of the body have a relation to the qualities of things external, and that delicacy of texture is a necessary consequence of this relation.

Wonderful, and exquisitely constructed, as the mechanical appliances are for the protection of this delicate structure, they are altogether insufficient ; and a protection of a very different kind, which shall animate the body to the utmost exertion, is requisite for safety. Pain, whilst it is a necessary contrast to its opposite pleasure, is the great safeguard of the frame. Finally, as to man, we shall be led to infer that the pains and pleasures of mere bodily sense (with yet more benevolent intention) carry us onward, through the developement and improvement of the mind itself, to higher aspirations.

Such is the course of reasoning which I propose to follow in giving an account of the hand and arm, contrasting them with the corresponding parts of living creatures, through all the divisions of the chain of vertebrated animals.

When I first thought of extending my notes on this subject, it appeared to me that I might have many other topics more prolific in proofs of design, and more interesting; but I now find that there is no end to illustration, and that the subject branches out interminably.

Some may conceive that as I have for my title the Human Hand, and the relation of the solid structures of the animal frame, it will lead me to consider the body as a machine only. I neither see the necessity for this, nor do I acknowledge the danger of considering it in that light. I embark fearlessly in the investigation, convinced that, yielding to the current of thought, and giving the fullest scope to enquiry, there can be no hidden danger if the mind be free from vicious bias. I cannot see how scepticism should arise out of the contemplation of the structure and mechanism of the animal body.

Let us for a moment think what is the natural result of examining the human body as a piece of machinery, and let us see whether it makes the creation of man more or less important in his relation to the whole scheme of nature.

Suppose that there is placed before us a machine for raising great weights, be it the simplest of all, the wheel and axle. We are given to understand that this piece of mechanism has the property of multiplying the power of the hand. But a youth of subtile mind may say, I do not believe that it is possible so to multiply the power of the hand; and if the mechanician be a philosopher, he will rather applaud the spirit of doubt. If he condescend to explain, he will say, that the piles driven into the ground, or the screws which unite the machinery to the beams, are the fixed points which resist in the working of the machine; that their resistance is a necessary condition, since it is thrown, together with the power of the hand, on the weight to be raised. And he will add that the multiplication of wheels does not alter the principle of action, which every one may see in the simple lever, to result from the resistance of the fulcrum or point, on which it rests.

Now grant that man's body is a machine, where are the points of resistance? are they not in the ground he stands upon? This leads us to enquire by what property we stand. Is it by the weight of the body, or in other words, is it by the attraction of the earth? The terms attraction, or gravitation, lead at once to the philosophy of the question. We stand because the body has weight, and a resistance, in proportion to the matter of the animal frame, and the magnitude of the globe itself. We wait not at present to observe the adjustment of the strength of the frame, the resistance of the bones, the elasticity of the joints, and the power of the muscles to the weight of the whole. Our attention is directed to the relations which the frame has to the earth we are placed upon.

Some philosophers, who have considered the matter curiously, have said, that if man were translated bodily to another planet, and were it smaller than the earth, he would be too light, and he would walk like one wading in deep water. If the planet were larger, the attraction of his body would make him feel as if his limbs were loaded with lead; nay, the attraction might be so great as to destroy the fabric of the body, crushing bones and all.*

However idle these fancies may be, there is no doubt that the animal frame is formed with a due relation to the earth we inhabit, and that the parts of the animal body, and we may say the strength of the

---

* The matter of Jupiter is as 330,600 to 1000 of our Earth. The diameter of Pallas is 80 miles; the Earth is 7,911 miles in diameter.

materials, have as certainly a correspondence with the weight, as the wheels and levers of a machine, or the scaffolding which sustains them, have relation to the force and velocity of the machinery, or the load that they are employed to raise.

The mechanism and organization of animals have been often brought forward for a different purpose from that for which I use them. We find it said, that it is incomprehensible that an all-powerful Being should manifest his will in this manner; that mechanical contrivance implies difficulties overcome: and how strange it is, they add, that the perceptions of the mind, which might have been produced by some direct means, or have arisen spontaneously, are received through an instrument so fine and complex as the eye;—and which requires the creation of the element of light, to enter the organ and to cause vision.

For my own part, I think it most natural to contemplate the subject quite differently. We perhaps presume too much, when we say, that light has been created for the purpose of vision. We are hardly entitled to pass over its properties as a chemical agent, its influence on the gases, and, in all probability on the atmosphere, its importance to vegetation, to the formation of the aromatic and volatile principles, and to fructification, its influence on the animal surface by invigorating the circulation, and imparting health. In relation to our present subject, it seems more rational to consider light as second only to attraction, in respect to its importance in nature, and as a link connecting systems of infinite remoteness.

To have a conception of this we must tutor our minds, and acquire some measure of the velocity of light, and of the space which it fills. It is not sufficient to say that it moves 200,000 miles in a second; for we can comprehend no such degree of velocity. If we are further informed that the earth is distant from the sun 95,000,000 of miles, and that light traverses the space in 8 minutes and 1-8th, it is but another way of affirming the inconceivable rapidity of its transmission. Astronomers, the power of whose minds affords us the very highest estimate of human faculties, the accuracy of whose calculations is hourly visible to us, have affirmed that light emanates from celestial bodies at such vast distance, that thousands of years shall elapse during its progress to our earth: yet matter impelled by a force equal to its transmission through this space, shall enter the eye, and strike upon the delicate nerve with no other effect than to produce vision.

Instead of saying that light is created for the eye, and to give us the sense of vision, is it not more conformable to a just manner of considering these things that our wonder and our admiration should fix on the fact, that this small organ, the eye, is formed with relation to a creation of such vast extent and grandeur:—and more especially, that the ideas arising in the mind through the influence of that matter and this organ, are constituted a part of this vast whole !

By such considerations we are led to contemplate the human body in its different relations. The magnitude of the earth determines the strength of our bones, and the power of our muscles; so must the depth of the atmosphere determine the condition of our fluids, and the resistance of our blood vessels; the common act of breathing, the transpiration from the surfaces, must bear relation to the weight, moisture, and temperature of the medium which surrounds us. A moment's reflection on these facts proves to us that our body is formed with a just correspondence to all these external influences.

These views lead us to another consideration, that the complexity of our structure belongs to external nature, and not of necessity to the mind. Whilst man is an agent in a material world, and sensible to the influence of things external, complexity of structure is a necessary part of his constitution. But we do not perceive a relation between this complexity

and the mind. From aught that we learn by this
mode of study, the mind may be as distinct from the
bodily organs as are the exterior influences which give
them exercise.

Something, then, we observe to be common to our
planet and to others, to our system and to other systems; matter, attraction, light; which nearly implies
that the mechanical and chemical laws must be the
same throughout. It is perhaps too much to affirm,
with an anonymous author, that an inhabitant of our
world would find himself at home in any other, that
he would be like a traveller only, for a moment per-
plexed by diversity of climate and strangeness of man-
ners, and confess, at last, that nature was every where
and essentially the same. However this may be, all
I contend for is, the necessity of certain relations being
established between the planet and the frames of all
which inhabit it; between the great mass and the
physical properties of every part; that in the mechanical construction of animals, as in their endowments
of life, they are created in relation to the whole, planned
together and fashioned by one Mind.

The passiveness which is natural in infancy, and
the want of reflection as to the sources of enjoyment
which is excusable in youth, become insensibility and
ingratitude in riper years. In the early stages of life,
before our minds have the full power of comprehension, the objects around us serve but to excite and
exercise the outward senses. But in the maturity of
reason, philosophy should present these things to us
anew, with this difference, that the mind may contemplate them : that mind which is now strengthened by
experience to comprehend them, and to entertain a
grateful sense of them.

It is this sense of gratitude which distinguishes man.
In brutes, the attachment to offspring for a limited
period is as strong as in him, but it ceases with the
necessity for it. In man, on the contrary the affections

continue, become the sources of all the endearing relations of life, and the very bonds by which society is connected.

If the child, upon the parent's knee, is unconsciously incurring a debt, and strong affections grow up so naturally that nothing is more universally condemned than filial ingratitude, we have but to change the object of affection, to find the natural source of religion itself. We must show that the care of the most tender parent is in nothing to be compared with those provisions for our enjoyment and safety, which it is not only beyond the ingenuity of man to provide, but which he can hardly comprehend, while he profits by them.

If man, of all living creatures, be alone capable of gratitude, and through this sense be capable also of religion, the transition is natural; since the gratitude due to parents is abundantly more owing to Him "who "saw him in his blood, and said, Live."

For the continuance of life, a thousand provisions are made. If the vital actions of a man's frame were directed by his will, they are necessarily so minute and complicated, that they would immediately fall into confusion. He cannot draw a breath, without the exercise of sensibilities as well ordered as those of the eye or ear. A tracery of nervous cords unites many organs in sympathy, of which, if one filament were broken, pain and spasm, and suffocation would ensue. The action of his heart, and the circulation of his blood, and all the vital functions are governed through means and by laws which are not dependant on his will, and to which the powers of his mind are altogether inadequate. For had they been under the influence of his will, a doubt, a moment's pause of irresolution, a forgetfulness of a single action at its appointed time, would have terminated his existence.

Now, when man sees that his vital operations could not be directed by reason—that they are constant, and far too important to be exposed to all the changes

incident to his mind, and that they are given up to
the direction of other sources of motion than the will,
he acquires a full sense of his dependance.   If man
be fretful and wayward, and subject to inordinate passion, we perceive the benevolent design in withdraw-
ing the vital motions from the influence of such capri-
cious sources of action, so that they may neither be
disturbed like his moral actions, nor lost in a moment
of despair.

Ray, in speaking of the first drawing of breath,
delivers himself very naturally :   " Here, methinks,
" appears a necessity of bringing in the agency or
" some superintendant intelligent being, for what else
" should put the diaphragm and the muscles serving
" respiration in motion all of a sudden so soon as ever
" the fœtus is brought forth ? Why could they not
" have rested as well as they did in the womb ?
" What aileth them that they must needs bestir them-
" selves to get in air to maintain the creature's life ?
" Why could they not patiently suffer it to die ? You
" will say the spirits do at this time flow to the or-
" gans of respiration, the diaphragm, and other mus-
" cles which concur to that action and move them.
" But what raises the spirits which were quiescent,
" &c., I am not subtile enough to discover."

We cannot call this agency, a new intelligence
different from the mind, because, independently of
consciousness, we can hardly so define it. But there
is bestowed a sensibility, which being roused (and it is
excited by the state of the circulation,) governs these
muscles of respiration, and ministers to life and safety,
independently of the will.

When man thus perceives, that in respect to all
these vital operations he is more helpless than the
infant, and that his boasted reason can neither give
them order nor protection, is not his insensibility to the
Giver of these secret endowments worse than ingratitude ? In a rational creature, ignorance of his condition becomes a species of ingratitude ; it dulls his sense

of benefits, and hardens him into a temper of mind with which it is impossible to reason, and from which no improvement can be expected.

Debased in some measure by a habit of inattention, and lost to all sense of the benevolence of the Creator, he is roused to reflection only by overwhelming calamities, which appear to him magnified and disproportioned ; and hence arises a conception of the Author of his being more in terror than in love.

There is inconsistency and something of the child's propensities still in mankind. A piece of mechanism, as a watch, a barometer, or a dial, will fix attention— a man will make journeys to see an engine stamp a coin, or turn a block ; yet the organs through which he has a thousand sources of enjoyment, and which are in themselves more exquisite in design and more curious both in contrivance and in mechanism, do not enter his thoughts ; and if he admire a living action, that admiration will probably be more excited by what is uncommon and monstrous, than by what is natural and perfectly adjusted to its office—by the elephant's trunk, than by the human hand. This does not arise from an unwillingness to contemplate the superiority or dignity of our own nature, nor from an incapacity of admiring the adaptation of parts. It is the effect of habit. The human hand is so beautifully formed, it has so fine a sensibility, that sensibility governs its motions so correctly, every effort of the will is answered so instantly, as if the hand itself were the seat of that will ; its actions are so powerful, so free, and yet so delicate, that it seems to possess a quality instinct in itself, and there is no thought of its complexity as an instrument, or of the relations which make it subservient to the mind ; we use it as we draw our breath, unconsciously, and have lost all recollection of the feeble and ill-directed efforts of its first exercise, by which it has been perfected. Is it not the very perfection of the instrument which makes us insensible to its use ? A vulgar admiration is excited by seeing the spider-monkey pick up a straw, or a piece of wood, with its tail ; or the elephant searching the keeper's pocket with his trunk. Now, fully to examine the peculiarity of the elephant's structure, that is to say, from its huge mass, to deduce the necessity for its form, and from the form the necessity for its trunk, would lead us through a train of very curious observations, to a more correct notion of that appendage, and therefore to a truer admiration of it. But I take this part in contrast with the human hand, merely to show how insensible we are to the perfections of our own frame, and to the advantages attained through such a form. We use the limbs without being conscious, or, at least, without any conception of the thousand parts which must conform to a single act. To excite our attention, we must either see the actions of the human frame performed in some mode, strange and unexpected, such as may raise the wonder of the ignorant and vulgar ; or by an effort of the cultivated mind, we must rouse ourselves to observe things and actions, of which, as we have said, the sense has been lost by long familiarity.

In the following essay, I shall take up the subject comparatively, and exhibit a view of the bones of the arm, descending from the human hand to the fin of the fish.   I shall in the next place review the actions of the muscles of the arm and hand ; then proceeding to the vital properties, I shall advance to the subject of sensibility, leading to that of touch; afterwards, I shall show the necessity of combining the muscular action with the exercise of the senses, and especially with that of touch, to constitute in the hand what has been called the geometrical sense.

I shall describe the organ of touch, the cuticle and skin, and arrange the nerves of the hand according to their functions.   I shall then enquire into the correspondence between the capacities and endowments of the mind, in comparison with the external organs, and more especially with the properties of the hand ; and conclude by showing that animals have been created with a reference to the globe they inhabit ; that all their endowments and various organization bear a relation to their state of existence, and to the elements around them ; that there is a plan universal, extending through all animated nature, and which has prevailed in the earliest condition of the world ; and that, finally, in the most minute or most comprehensive study of those things we every where see prospective design.

CHAPTER II.

WE ought to define the hand as belonging exclusively to man—corresponding in sensibility and motion with that ingenuity which converts the being who is the weakest in natural defence, to the ruler over animate and inanimate nature.

If we describe the hand as that extremity which has the thumb and fingers opposed to each other, so as to form an instrument of prehension, we extend it to the quadrumana or monkeys. But the possession of four hands by animals of that class implies that we include the posterior as well as the anterior extremities. Now the anterior extremity of the monkey is as much a foot as the posterior extremity is a hand; both are calculated for their mode of progression, climbing, and leaping from the branches of trees, just as the tail in some species is converted into a hand, and is as useful an instrument of suspension as any of the four extremities.*

The armed extremities of a variety of animals give them great advantages; but if man possessed any

---

* The Coaita, or Spider Monkey, so called from the extraordinary length of its extremities, and its motions. The tail answers all the purposes of a hand, and the animal throws itself about from branch to branch, sometimes swinging from the foot, sometimes by the hand, but oftener and with a greater reach by the tail. The prehensile part of the tail is covered only with skin, forming an organ of touch, as discriminating as the hand. The Caraya, or Black howling monkey of Cumana, when shot, is found suspended by its tail, round a branch. Naturalists have been so struck with the property of the tail of the Ateles, as to compare it with the proboscis of the elephant; they have assured us that they fish with it.

The most interesting use of the tail is seen in the Opossum. The young of that animal entwine their tails around their mother's tail and mount upon her back, where they sit secure, while she escapes from her enemies.

similar provisions, he would forfeit his sovereignty over all. As Galen, long since, observed, "did man " possess the natural armour of the brutes, he would no ' longer work as an artificer, nor protect himself with a " breast-plate, nor fashion a sword or spear, nor invent " a bridle to mount the horse and hunt the lion. Nei- " ther could he follow the arts of peace, construct the " pipe and lyre, erect houses, place altars, inscribe laws, " and through letters hold communion with the wis- " dom of antiquity:"—"*tibique liceat literarum et ma-* " *nuum beneficiis etiam nunc colloqui cum Platone, cum-* " *Aristotele, cum Hippocrate.*"

But the hand is not a distinct instrument; nor is it properly a superadded part. The whole frame must conform to the hand, and act with reference to it. Our purpose will not be answered by examining it alone; we must extend our views to all those parts of the body which are in strict connection with the hand. For example, the bones from the shoulder to the fin- ger ends, have that systematic arrangement which makes it essential to examine the whole extremity; and in order fully to comprehend the fine arrange- ment of the parts, which is necessary to the motions of the fingers, we must also compare the structure of the human body with that of other animals.

Were we to limit our enquiry to the bones of the arm and hand in man, no doubt we should soon dis- cover their provisions for easy, varied, and powerful action; and conclude that nothing could be more perfectly suited to their purposes. But we must ex- tend our views to comprehend a great deal more,—a greater design.

By a skeleton, is understood the system of bones, which being internal, gives the characteristic form to the animal, and receives the action of the exterior muscles. This system belongs, however, only to one part of the animal kingdom, that higher division,—the animalia vertebrata, which includes the whole chain of beings, from man to fishes.

The function of the greatest consequence to life is respiration ; and the mode in which this is performed, that is to say, the manner in which the decarbonization of the blood is effected through its exposure to the atmosphere, produces a remarkable change in the whole frame-work of the animal body.

Man, the mammalia, birds, reptiles, and fishes have much of the mechanism of respiration in common ; and there is a resemblance through them all, in the texture of the bones, in the action of the muscles, and in the arrangement of the nerves. They all possess the vertebral column or spine ; and the existence of this column, not only implies an internal skeleton, but that particular frame-work of ribs, which is suited to move in breathing. But the ribs do not move of themselves, they must have appropriate muscles; and these muscles must have their appropriate nerves; and for supplying these nerves there must be a spinal marrow. The spinal canal is as necessary to the spinal marrow as the skull is to the brain. So that we come round to understand the necessity of a vertebra, to the formation of the spinal marrow ; and the reader may comprehend how much enters into the conception of the anatomist or naturalist, when the term is used, a vertebrated animal, viz :—an internal skeleton, a particular arrangement of respiratory organs, and a conformity in the nervous system.

It is to this superior division that I shall limit myself, in making a review of the bones of the upper extremity.

Were I to indulge in the admiration naturally arising out of this subject, and point out the strength and the freedom of motion in the upper extremity at the ball and socket joint of the shoulder,—the firmness of the articulation of the elbow, and yet how admirably it is suited to the co-operation of the hands,—the fineness of the motion of the hand itself, divided among the joints of twenty-nine bones, it might be objected to with some show of reason ; and it might be said, the bones and the forms of the joints which you are admiring, are so far from being peculiarly suited to the hand of man, that they may be found in any other vertebrated animal.

But this would not abate our admiration, it would only induce us to take a more comprehensive view of nature, and remind us that our error was in looking at a part only, instead of embracing the whole system; where by slight changes and gradations hardly perceptible, the same bones are adjusted to every condition of animal existence.

We recognize the bones which form the upper extremity of man, in the fin of the whale, in the paddle of the turtle, and in the wing of the bird. We see the same bones, perfectly suited to their purpose, in the paw of the lion or the bear, and equally fitted for motion in the hoof of the horse, or in the foot of the camel, or adjusted for climbing or digging in the long clawed feet of the sloth or bear.

It is obvious, then, that we should be occupied with too limited a view of our subject, were we to consider the human hand in any other light than as presenting the most perfect combination of parts: as exhibiting the parts, which in different animals are suited to particular purposes, so combined in the hand, as to perform actions the most minute and complicated, consistently with powerful exertion.

The wonder still is, that whether we examine this system in man, or in any of the inferior species of animals, nothing can be more curiously adjusted or appropriated; and we should be inclined to say, whatever instance occupied our thoughts for the time, that to this particular object the system had been framed.

The view which the subject opens to us, is unbounded. The curous synthesis by which we ascertain the nature, condition, and habits of an extinct animal, from the examination of its fossil remains, is grounded on a knowledge of the system of which we are speaking. A bone consists of many parts; but for our present purpose it is only necessary to observe that the hard substance, the phosphate of lime, which we familiarly recognize as bone, is every where penetrated by membranes and vessels as delicate as those which belong to any other part of the body. Some bones are found with their animal part remaining, others are fossilized. The phosphate of lime loses its phosphoric acid, and the earth of bone remains incorruptible, while the softer animal matter undergoes the process of decomposition, and is dissipated. The bone in this condition may become fossilized; silicious earth, or lime in composition with iron, or iron pyrites, may pass by infiltration into the interstices of the original earthy matter, and in this state it is as permanent as the solid rock. It retains the form, though not the internal structure of bone; and that form, in consequence of the perfect system which we have hinted at, becomes a proof of revolutions the most extraordinary. The mind of the enquirer is carried back, not merely to the contemplation of animal structure, but by inference, from the system of animal organization to the structure of the globe itself.

The bones of large animals and in great variety are found imbedded in the surface of the earth. They are discovered in the beds of rivers, they are found where no waters flow, they are dug up from under the solid limestone rock. The bones thus exposed, become naturally a subject of intense interest, and are unexpectedly connected with the enquiry in which we are engaged. Among other important conclusions they lead to this—that there is not only a scheme or system of animal structure pervading all the classes of animals which inhabit the earth, but that the principle of this great plan of creation was in operation, and governed the formation of those animals which existed previous to the revolutions that the earth itself has undergone: that the excellence of form now seen in the skeleton of man, was in the scheme of animal existence long previous to the formation of man, and before the surface of

the earth was prepared for him or suited to his constitution, structure, or capacities.

A skeleton is dug up which has lain under many
fathoms of rock : being the bones of an animal
which lived antecedent to that formation of rock, and .
at a time when the earth's surface must have been in
a condition very different from what it is now. These
remains prove, that all animals have been formed of
the same elements, and have had analogous organs
—that they received new matter by digestion, and
were nourished by means of a circulating fluid—that
they possessed feeling through a nervous system, and
were moved by the action of muscles—that their organs of digestion, circulation, and respiration were
modified by circumstances, as in the animals now alive,
and in accordance with their habits and modes of living.   The changes in the organs are but variations in
the great system by which new matter is assimilated
to the animal body,—and however remarkable these
may be, they always bear a certain. relation to the
original type as parts of the same great design.

In examining these bones of the ancient world, so
regularly are they formed on the same principle which
is evident in the animals now inhabiting the earth,
that on observing their shape, and the processes by
which their muscles were attached, we can reduce
the animals to which they belonged, to their orders,
genera, and species, with as much precision as if the recent bodies had been submitted to the eye of the anatomist.   Not only can we demonstrate that their feet
were adapted to the solid ground, or to the oozy bed
of rivers,—for speed, or for grasping and tearing ; but
judging by these indications of the habits of the animals, we acquire a knowledge of the condition of the
earth during their period of existence ; that it was
suited at one time to the scaly tribe of the lacertæ,
with languid motion ; at another, to animals of higher
organization, with more varied and lively habits ; and
finally we learn, that at any period previous to man's

creation, the surface of the earth would have been unsuitable to him.

On comparing some of the present races of animals, with the fossil remains of individuals of the same family, some singular opinions on their imperfections have been expressed by Buffon, and adopted by Cuvier. The animals I allude to are of the tardigrade family ; the Ai,* in which, as they believe, the defect of organizaton is the greatest ; and the Unau,† which they consider only a little less miserably provided for existence.

Modern travellers express their pity for these animals : whilst other quadrupeds, they say, range in boundless wilds, the sloth hangs suspended by his strong arms—a poor ill-formed creature, deficient as well as deformed, his hind legs too short, and his hair like withered grass ; his looks, motions, and cries conspire to excite pity ; and, as if this were not enough, they say that his moaning makes the tiger relent and turn away. This is not a true picture : the sloth cannot walk like quadrupeds, but he stretches out his strong arms,—and if he can hook on his claws to the inequalities of the ground, he drags himself along. This is the condition which authorizes such an expression as " the bungled and faulty composition of the sloth." But when he reaches the branch or the rough bark of a tree, his progress is rapid ; he climbs hand over head, along the branches till they touch, and thus from bough to bough, and from tree to tree ; he is most alive in the storm, and when the wind blows, and the trees stoop, and the branches wave and meet, he is then upon the march.

The compassion expressed by these philosophers for animals,‡ which they consider imperfectly organ-

* Bradypus Tridactylus :—bradypus (*slow footed,*) tridactylus (*three toed,*) of the order EDENTATA (*wanting incisor teeth.*)
† Bradypus didactylus.
‡ The subject is pursued in the end of the following chapter.

ized, is uncalled for ; as well might they pity the
larva of the summer fly, which creeps in the bottom
of a pool, because it cannot yet rise upon the wing.
As the insect has no impulse to fly until the metamorphosis is perfect, and the wings developed, so we
have no reason to suppose that a disposition or instinct
is given to animals, where there is no corresponding
provision for motion.

The sloth may move tardily on the ground, his long
arms and his preposterous claws may be an incum-
brance, but they are of advantage in his natural place,
among the branches of trees, in obtaining his food,
and in giving him shelter and safety from his enemies.

We must not estimate the slow motions of animals
by our own sensations. The motion of the bill of the
swallow, or the fly-catcher, in catching a fly, is so rapid that we do not see it, but only hear the snap. On
the contrary, how very different are the means given
to the chamelion for obtaining his food; he lies more
still than the dead leaf, his skin is like the bark of
the tree, and takes the hue of surrounding objects.
Whilst other animals have excitement conforming to
their rapid motions, the shrivelled face of the chamelion hardly indicates life ; the eyelids are scarcely
parted ; he protrudes his tongue with a motion so
imperceptible towards the insect, that it is touched
and caught more certainly than by the most lively
action. Thus, various creatures living upon insects,
reach their prey by different means and instincts ;
rapidity of motion, which gives no time for escape, is
bestowed on some, while others have a languid and
slow movement that excites no alarm.

The loris, a tardigrade animal, might be pitied too
for the slowness of its motions, if they were not the
very means bestowed upon it as necessary to its
existence. It steals on its prey by night, and extends its arm to the bird on the branch, with a
motion so imperceptibly slow, as to make sure of its

object.*   Just so, the Indian perfectly naked, his hair
cut short, and his skin oiled, creeps under the canvass
of the tent, and moving like a ghost, stretches out his
hand, with so gentle a motion as to displace nothing,
and to disturb not even those who are awake and
watching.   Against such thieves, we are told, that it
is hardly possible to guard ; and thus, the necessities
or vicious desires of man subjugate him, and make
him acquire, by practice, the wiliness which is implanted as instinct in brutes ; or we may say that
in our reason we are brought to imitate the irrational
creatures, and so to vindicate the necessity for their
particular instincts, of which every class affords an
instance.   We have examples in insects, as striking
as in the loris or the chamelion.   Evelyn describes
the actions of the spider (*aranea scenica*) as exhibiting
remarkable cunning in catching a fly.   "Did the
" fly, (he says,) happen not to be within a leap, the
" spider would move towards it, so softly, that its
" motion seemed not more perceptible than that of
" the shadow of the gnomon of a dial."†
    I would only remark further on these slow motions

---

* For our purpose, it may be well to notice other characters of this
and similar animals which prowl by night.   They are inhabitants of
the tropical regions.   Now, the various creatures which enliven the
woods in the day-time, in these warm climates, have fine skins, and
smooth hair; but those have a coat like animals of the arctic regions.
What is this, but to clothe them, as the sentinel is clothed, whose
watch is in the night.   They have eyes too, which, from their peculiarity, are called nocturnal, being formed to admit a greater pencil of rays.
For this purpose the globe is large and prominent, and the iris contractile, to open the pupil to the greatest extent.—We have seen
how all their motions and instincts correspond with their nocturnal
habits.

† The passage continues—"if the intended prey moved, the spider
would keep pace with it exactly as if they were actuated by one spirit,
moving backwards, forwards, or on each side without turning.   When
the fly took wing, and pitched itself behind the huntress, she turned
round with the swiftness of thought, and always kept her head towards it, though to all appearance as immoveable as one of the nails
driven into the wood on which was her station; till at last, being arrived within due distance, swift as lightning she made the fatal leap,
and secured her prey."—Evelyn, as quoted by Kirby and Spence.

of the muscles of animals; that we are not to account this a defect, but rather an appropriation of muscular power. Since in some animals the same muscles which move their members in a manner to be hardly perceptible, can at another time act with the velocity of a spring.

Now Buffon, speaking of the extinct species of the tardigrade family, considers them as monsters by defect of organization; as attempts of nature in which she has failed to perfect her plan; that she has produced animals which must have lived miserably, and which are effaced as failures from the list of living beings. The Baron Cuvier does not express himself more favorably, when he says of the existing species, that they have so little resemblance to the organization of animals generally, and their structure is so much in contrast with that of other creatures, that he could believe them to be the remnants of an order unsuitable to the present system of nature; and if we are to look for their congeners, it must be in the interior of the earth, in the ruins of the ancient world.

The animals of the Antediluvian world were not monsters; there was no lusus or extravagance. Hideous as they appear to us, and like the phantoms of a dream, they were adapted to the condition of the earth when they existed. I could have wished that our naturalists had given the inhabitants of that early condition of the globe, names less scholastic. We have the plesiosaurus, and plesiosaurus dolichodeirus, we have the ichthyosaurus and megalosaurus, and iguanodon, pterodactyles, with long and short beaks, tortoises, and crocodiles; and these are found among reeds and grasses of gigantic proportions, algæ and fuci, and a great variety of mollusca of inordinate bulk, compared with those of the present day, as ammonites and nautili. Every thing declares, that these animals inhabited shallow seas, and estuaries, or great inland lakes: that the surface of the earth did not rise up in peaks and mountains, or that perpendicular rocks bound in the seas; but that it was flat, slimy, and covered with a loaded and foggy atmosphere. There is, indeed, every reason to believe that the classes mammalia and birds were not then created, and that if man had been placed in this condition of the earth, there must have been around him a state of things unsuited to his constitution, and not calculated to call forth his capacities.

But looking to the class of animals as we have enumerated them, there is a correspondence; they were scaly; they swam in water, or crept upon the margins; there were no animals possessed of rapidity of motion, and no birds of prey to stoop upon them; there was, in short, that balance of the power of destruction and of self preservation, which we see now to obtain in higher animals since created, with infinitely varied instincts and powers for defence or attack.

It is hardly possible to watch the night and see the break of day in a fine country, without being sensible that our pleasantest perceptions refer to the scenery of nature, and that we have feelings in sympathy with every successive change, from the first streak of light, until the whole landscape is displayed in valleys, woods, and sparkling waters; and the changes on the scene are not more rapid than the transitions of the feelings which accompany them. All these sources of enjoyment, the clear atmosphere and the refreshing breezes, are as certainly the result of the several changes which the earth's surface has undergone, as the displaced strata within its crust are demonstrative of these changes. We have every reason to conclude that these revolutions, whether they have been slowly accomplished and progressively or by sudden, vast and successive convulsions, were necessary to prepare the earth for that condition which should correspond with the faculties to be given to man, and be suited to the full exercise of his reason, as well as to his enjoyment.

If a man contemplate the common objects around him—if he observe the connection between the qualities of things external and the exercise of his senses, between the senses so excited, and the condition of his mind, he will perceive that he is in the centre of a magnificent system, and that the strictest relation is established between the intellectual capacities and the material world.

In the succeeding chapter we shall take a comparative view of the anatomy of the arm, and we shall be led to observe some very extraordinary changes, as we trace the same parts through different genera and species of animals. In doing this, we are naturally called upon to notice certain opinions which prevail on the subject.

We have already hinted, that geologists have discovered, that in the stratified rocks there is proof of a regular succession of formations in the crust of the earth, and that animals of very different structure have been imbedded, and are preserved in them. In the earlier formed strata animals are found which are low, as we choose to express it, in the chain of existence; in higher strata, oviparous animals of great bulk, and more complex structure, are discovered; above the strata containing these oviparous reptiles, there are found mammalia; and in the looser and more superficial stratum are the bones of the mastodon, megatherium, rhinoceros, and elephant, &c. We must add that geologists agree that man has been created last of all.

Upon these facts, a theory is raised, that there has been a succession of animals gradually increasing in the perfection of their structure; that the first impulse of nature was not sufficient to the production of the highest and most perfect, and that it was only in her mature efforts that mammalia were produced. We are led to this reflection: that the creation of a living animal, the bestowing of life on a

4

corporeal frame, however simple the structure of that
body, is of itself, an act of creative power so inconceivably great, that we can have no title to presume
that the change in the organization, such as the
provision of bones and muscles, or the production of
new organs of sense, is a higher effort of that power.
We have a better guide in exploring the varieties of
animated nature, when we acknowledge the manifest design with which all is accomplished; the
adaptation of the animals, their size, their economy,
their organs, and instruments to their condition.

Whether we make the most superficial or most
profound examination of animals in their natural
state, we shall find that the varieties are so balanced
as to ensure the existence of all. This, we think,
goes far to explain, first, why the remains of certain
animals are found in certain strata, which imply a
peculiar condition of the earth's surface; and, secondly, why these animals are found grouped together. For, as we may express it, if there had been
an error in the grouping, there must have been a
destruction of the whole; the balance which is necessary to their existence having been destroyed.
We know very well that so minute a thing as a fly,
will produce, in twenty-four hours, millions, which,
if not checked, will ere long darken the air, and render whole regions desolate; so that if the breeze does
not carry them in due time into the desert, or into the
ocean, the destruction will be most fearful.

As in the present day every creature has its natural
enemy; or is checked in production, sometimes by a
limited supply of food, sometimes by disease, or by the
influence of seasons; and as in the whole a balance is
preserved, we may reasonably apply the same principle in explanation of the condition of things as they
existed in the earlier stages of the world's progress;
certainly, this view is borne out, by what we have as
yet discovered in the grouping of animals, in the
different stratifications or deposits of the earth.

If the naturalist or geologist, exploring the rocks of secondary formation, should find inclosed within them animals of the class Molusca, it agrees with his preconceived notions, that only animals of their simple structure were in existence, at the time of the subsidence of that matter of which the rock consists. But if the spine of a fish, or a jawbone, or a tooth, be discovered, he is much disturbed, because, here is the indication of an animal having been at that time formed on a different type,—on that plan which belongs to animals of a superior class.—Whereas on the supposition that animals are created with that relation to circumstances, which we have just alluded to, it would only imply that certain animals, which had hitherto increased undisturbed, had arrived at a period, when their numbers were to be limited; or that the condition of the elements and the abundance of food were now suited to the existence of a species of the vertebrata.

The principle then, in the application of which we shall be borne out, is, that there is an adaptation, an established and universal relation between the instincts, organization, and instruments of animals on the one hand, and the element in which they are to live, the position which they hold, and their means of obtaining food on the other;—and this holds good with respect to the animals which have existed, as well as those which now exist.

In discussing this subject of the progressive improvement of organized beings, it is affirmed that the last created of all, man, is not superior in organization to the others, and that if deprived of intellectual power he is inferior to the brutes. I am not arguing to support the gradual developement and improvement of organization; but, however indifferent to the tendency of the argument, I must not admit the statement. Man is superior in organization to the brutes,—superior in strength—in that constitutional property which enables him to fulfil his destinies by extending his race in every climate, and living on every variety of nutriment. Gather together the most powerful brutes, from the artic circle or torrid zone, to some central point—they will die, diseases will be generated, and will destroy them. With respect to the superiority of man being in his mind, and not merely in the provisions of his body, it is no doubt true ;—but as we proceed, we shall find how the Hand supplies all instruments, and by its correspondence with the intellect gives him universal dominion. It presents the last and best proof of that principle of adaptation, which evinces design in the creation.

Another notion which we meet with. is, that the variety of animals is not a proof of design, as showing a relation between the formation of their organs, and the necessity for their exercise ; but that the circumstances in which the animal has been placed, have been the cause of the variety. The influence of these circumstances, it is pretended, has, in the long progress of time, produced a complication of structure out of an animal which was at first simple. We shall reserve the discussion of this subject until we have the data before us ; which, of themselves, and without much argument, will suffice to overthrow it. I may notice here another idea of naturalists, who are pleased to reduce these changes in the structure of animals into general laws. They affirm that in the centre of the animal body there is no disposition to change, whilst in the extremities we see surprising variations of form. If this be a law, there is no more to be said about it, the enquiry is terminated. But I contend that the term is quite inapplicable, and worse than useless, as tending to check enquiry. What then is the meaning of this variation in the extremities and comparative permanence towards the centre of the skeleton ? I conceive the rationale to be this, that the central part, by which in fact they mean the skull, spine, and ribs, are permanent in their offices ; whilst the extremities vary and are adapted to every exterior circumstance. The office of the back part of the skull is to protect the brain, that of the spine to contain the spinal marrow, and the ribs to perform respiration. Why should we expect these parts to vary in shape while their office remains the same? But the shoulder must vary in form, as it does in motion. The shape of the bones and the joints of the extremities must be adapted to their various actions, and the carpus and phalanges must change, more than all the rest, to accommodate the extremity to its different offices. Is it not more pleasing to see the reason of this most surprising adjustment, than merely to say it is a law?

There is yet another opinion, which will suggest itself by the perusal of the following chapter, to those who have read the more modern works on Natural History. It is supposed that the same elementary parts belong to all animals, and that the varieties of structure are attributable to the transposition and moulding of these elementary parts. I find it utterly impossible to follow up this system to the extent which its abettors would persuade us to be practicable. I object to it as a means of engaging us in very trifling pursuits,—and of diverting the mind from the truth ; from that conclusion, indeed, to which I may avow it to be my intention to carry the reader. But this discussion also must follow the examples, and we shall resume it in a latter part of the volume.

CHAPTER III.

THE COMPARATIVE ANATOMY OF THE HAND.

In this enquiry, we have before us what in the strictest sense of the word is a system. All the individuals of the extensive division of the animal kingdom which we have to review, possess a cranium for the protection of the brain,—a heart, implying a peculiar circulation,—five distinguishable organs of sense; but the grand peculiarity, whence the term vertebrata is derived, is to be found in the spine; that chain of bones which connects the head and body, and, like a keel, serves as a foundation for the ribs; or as the basis of that fabric which is for respiration.

I have said, that we are to confine ourselves to a portion only of this combined structure; to separate and examine the anterior extremity, and to observe the adaptation of its parts, through the whole range of these animals. We shall view it as it exists in man, and in the higher division of animals which give suck, the mammalia—in those which propagate by eggs, the oviparous animals,—birds, reptiles, amphibia, and fishes; and we shall find the bones which are identified by distinct features, adjusted to various purposes, in all the series, from the arm to the fin. We shall recognize them in the mole, formed into a powerful apparatus for digging, by which the animal soon covers itself, and burrows its way under ground. In the wing of the eagle we shall count every bone adapted to a new element, and as powerful to rise in the air, as the fin of the salmon is to strike through the water. The solid hoof of the horse, the cleft foot of the ruminant, the retractile claw of the feline tribe, the long folding nails of the sloth, are among the many changes that are found in the adjustment of the chain of bones which, in man, ministers to the compound motions of the hand.

OF THE SHOULDER.

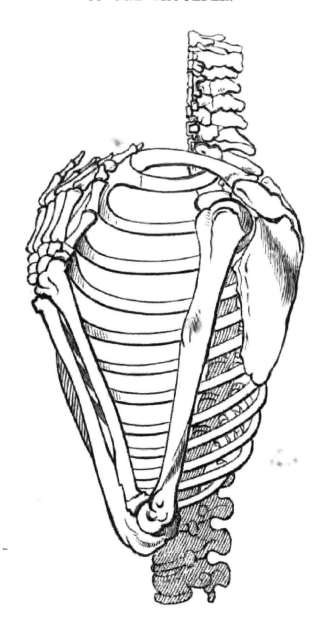

Were it my purpose to teach the elements of this subject, I should commence with examining the lowest animals, and trace the bones of the anterior extremity as they come to resemble the human arm, and to be employed for a greater variety of uses in the higher animals; but as my present object is illustration only, I shall begin with the human hand, and compare its parts. With this view, I shall divide the extremity into the shoulder, arm, and hand, and treat each subdivision with a reference to its structure in animals.

In viewing the human figure, or human skeleton, in connection with our present subject, we remark the strength and solidity of the lower extremities, in contrast with the superior. Not only are the lower limbs longer and larger than those of any other animal, but the pelvis is wider, and the obliquity of the neck of the thigh-bone greater. The distances of the large processes on the upper ends of the thigh-bones (the trochanters,) from the sockets, are also greater than in any of the vertebrata. Altogether the strength of these bones, the size and prominence of their processes, the great mass of the muscles of the loins and hips, distinguish man from every other animal; they secure to him the upright posture, and give him the perfect freedom of the arms, for purposes of ingenuity and art.

The Chimpanzee* is an ape which stands high in

---

* *Simia troglodytes,* from the coast of Guinea, more human in its form, and more easily domesticated than the ourang-outang. We would do well to consider the abode of these creatures in a state of nature—vast forests extending in impenetrable shade below, whilst above, and exposed to the light, there is a scene of verdure and beauty; this is the home of those monkeys and lemurs which have extremities like hands. In many of them the hinder extremity has the more perfect resemblance to a hand; in the Coaita we see the great toe assuming the characters of a thumb, whilst in the fore paw, the thumb is not distinguishable, being hid in the skin. In short, these paws are not approximations to the hand, corresponding with a higher ingenuity, but are adaptations of the feet to the branches on which the animals climb.

the order of quadrumana, yet we cannot mistake his capacities : that the lower extremities and pelvis, or hips, were never intended to give him the erect posture, or only for a moment ; but, for swinging, or for a vigorous pull, who can deny him power in those long and sinewy arms.

The full prominent shoulders, and the consequent squareness of the trunk, are equally distinctive of man, with the strength of his loins; they indicate a free motion of the hand.

OF THE BONES OF THE SHOULDER.

The bones of the shoulder, being those which give firm attachment to the upper extremity, and which afford origins to the muscles of the arm and fore arm, are simple, if studied in man, or, indeed, in any one genus of animals ; but considered in reference to the whole of the vertebral animals, they assume a very extraordinary degree of intricacy. We shall, however, find that they retain their proper office, notwithstanding the strange variations in the form of the neighbouring parts. In man they are directly connected with the great apparatus of respiration ; but in other animals we shall see the ribs, as it were, withdrawn from them, and the bones of the shoulder, or fundamental bones of the extremity, curiously and mechanically adapted to perform their office, without the support of the thorax. We shall not, however, anticipate the difficulties of this subject, but look first upon that which is most familiar and easy, the shoulder of man in comparison with the varieties in the mammalia.

The *clavicle*, or collar bone, is that which runs across from the breast bone to the top of the shoulder. The square form of the chest, and the free exercise of the hand, are very much owing to this bone. It keeps the shoulders apart from the chest, and throws

the action of the muscles upon the arm bone, which,
but for it, would be drawn inwards, and contract the
upper part of the trunk.

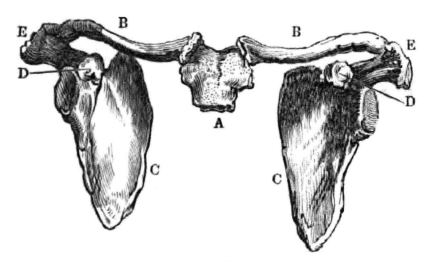

If we take the motions of the anterior extremity
in different animals, as our guide, we shall see why
this bone is perfect in some, and entirely wanting in
others.   Animals which fly, or dig, or climb, as bats,
moles, porcupines, squirrels, ant-eaters, armadilloes,
and sloths, have this bone, for in them, a lateral or
outward motion is required.   There is also a certain
degree of freedom in the anterior extremity of the
cat, dog, martin, and bear; they strike with the paw,
and rotate the wrist more or less extensively, and
they have therefore a clavicle, though an imperfect
one.   In some of these, even in the lion, the bone
which has the place of the clavicle is very imperfect
indeed; and if attached to the shoulder, it does not
extend to the sternum; it is concealed in the flesh,
and is like the mere rudiments of the bone.   But,
however imperfect, it marks a correspondence in the

A. Triangular portion of the Sternum.   B. B. Clavicles.   c. c.
Scapulæ.   D. Coracoid process of the Scapula.   E. Acromion process of the Scapulæ.

bones of the shoulder to those of the arm and paw, and the extent of motion enjoyed.

When the bear stands up, we perceive, by his ungainly attitude and the motion of his paws, that there must be a wide difference in the bones of his upper extremity, from those of the ruminant or solipede. He can take the keeper's hat from his head, and hold it; he can hug an animal to death. The ant-bear especially, as he is deficient in teeth, possesses extraordinary powers of hugging with his great paws; and, although harmless in disposition, he can squeeze his enemy, the jaguar, to death. These actions, and the power of climbing, result from the structure of the shoulder, or from possessing a collar bone, however imperfect.

Although the clavicle is perfect in man, thereby corresponding with the extent and freedom of the motion of his hand, it is strongest and longest, comparatively, in the animals which dig or fly, as in the mole and the bat.

Preposterous as the forms of the kangaroo appear to us, yet even in this animal we see a relation preserved between the extremities. He sits upon his strong hind legs and tail, tripod like, with perfect security, and his fore paws are free. He has a clavicle, and possessing that bone and the corresponding motions, is not without means of defence; for with the anterior extremities he seizes the most powerful dog, and then drawing up his hinder feet, he digs his sharp pointed hoofs into his enemy, and striking out, tears him to pieces. Though possessed of no great speed, and without horns, teeth, or claws, and, as we should suppose, totally defenceless, nature has not been negligent of his protection.*

* There is in the form of the kangaroo, and especially in its skeleton, something incongruous, and in contrast with the usual shape of quadrupeds. The head, trunk, and fore paws, appear to be a portion of an animal, unnaturally joined to another of greater dimensions and strength. It is not easy to say what are, or what were, the exte-

It cannot be better shown, that the function or use of a part, determines its form, than by looking to the clavicle and scapula of the bird.

Three bones converge here, to the shoulder joint, the furculum, clavicle, and scapula; but none of these have the resemblance which their names would imply. The scapula is the long thin bone, like the blade of a knife; and the clavicle is that stronger portion of bone which is articulated with the breast bone : this leaves the furculum as a new part. Now I think, that the furculum, or fork bone, which in carving, we detach, after removing the wings of a fowl, corresponds with the form and place of the clavicle ; and if we so consider it, we may then take

rior relations corresponding with the very peculiar form of this animal; but the interior anatomy is accommodated, in a most remarkable manner, to the enormous hinder extremities.

The uterine system of the female is diminutive, and does not undergo the developement, which universally takes place in other animals. The young, instead of remaining within the mother for the period of gestation, become, by some extraordinary mode of expulsion, attached to the teats ; where they hang by the mouth, covered by an exterior pouch, until, from minute and shapeless things, they are matured to the degree in which the young of other animals are usually produced. The artery which supplies the milk glands, is the epigastric, a branch of the great artery of the thigh ; and in this curious manner is the provision for the young drawn from the great limbs of the mother,— certainly the part best enabled to supply it.

I think I perceive the reason of this very peculiar manner of bringing forth the young, to be in the form of the animal and its upright position. The argument would stand thus, were we here at liberty to discuss it :. 1. An upright position of the mother requires a pelvis of a peculiar and complex construction. 2. A pelvis, of this construction, requires that the form of the offspring shall accurately correspond, and that the anterior part of the foetus shall much exceed in size the posterior parts. 3. But the kangaroo is, in shape, the very reverse,—the head could not, consistently with the conformation of the whole animal, be larger than the hips and hinder extremities. 4. Nature has accomplished her work safely, and by the simplest means, by anticipating the period of the separation of the foetus, and providing for the growth of the offspring, exterior to the circle of bones through which its birth must take place. It will, perhaps, be objected to this reasoning, that the order *didelphis* (with a double womb) embraces animals which have no such remarkable disproportion in the hinder extremities.

the strong bone, commonly called the clavicle, as a process of the irregularly formed scapula. However this may be, what we have to admire in birds, is the mode in which the bones are fashioned, to strengthen the articulation of the shoulder, and to give extent of surface for the attachment of muscles.

Another peculiarity in birds is, that there is not an alternate motion of the wings ; their extremities, as we may continue to call them, move together in flying ; and, therefore, the clavicles are joined, forming the furculum.

OF THE SCAPULA.

If we attend to the scapula, or shoulder-blade, we shall better understand the influence of the bones of the shoulder, on the motions and speed of animals. The scapula is that flat triangular bone, which lying on the ribs, and cushioned with muscles, shifts and revolves with each movement of the arm. The muscles converge from all sides towards it, from the head, spine, ribs, and breast bone. These acting in succession, roll the scapula and toss the arm, in every direction. When the muscles combine in action, they fix the bone, and either raise the ribs in drawing breath, or give firmness to the whole frame of the trunk.

Before I remark further on the influence of the scapulæ on the motions of the arm, I shall give an instance in proof of a very important function which they perform. Hearing that there was a lad of fourteen years of age, born without arms, I sent for him. I found that indeed he had no arms, but he had clavicles and scapulæ. When I made this boy draw his breath, the shoulders were raised, that is to say, the scapulæ were drawn up, were fixed, and became the points from which the broad muscles of the chest diverged towards the ribs, to draw and expand them in respiration. We would do well to remember this double office of the scapula and its muscles, that

5

whilst it is the very foundation of the bones of the upper extremity, and never wanting in any animal that has the most remote resemblance to an arm, it is the centre and point d'appui of the muscles of respiration, and acts in that capacity, where there are no extremities at all !

We perceive, that it is only in certain classes of animals, that the scapula is joined to the trunk by bone, that is, through the medium of a clavicle ; and a slight depression on a process of the scapula, when discovered in a fossil state, will declare to the geologist, the class to which the animal belonged. For example, there are brought over to this country the bones of the Megatherium, an animal, which must have been as large as the elephant ; of the anterior extremity there is only the scapula ; and on the extremity of the process, which is called acromion, of that bone, there is a mark of the attachment of a clavicle. This points out the whole constitution of the extremity, and that it enjoyed perfect freedom of motion. Other circumstances will declare whether that extensive motion was bestowed, so that the animal might dig with its huge claws like some of the edentata, or strike like the feline tribe.

Some interest is attached to the position of the scapula, in the horse. In him, and in other quadrupeds, with the exceptions which I have made, there is no clavicle, and the connection between the extremity and the trunk, is solely through muscles. That muscle, called serratus magnus, which is a large one in man, is particularly powerful in the horse ; for the weight of the trunk hangs upon this muscle. In the horse, as in most quadrupeds, the speed results from the strength of the loins and hinder extremities, for it is the muscles there which propel the animal. But were the anterior extremities joined to the trunk firmly, and by bone, they could not withstand the shock from the descent of the whole weight thrown forwards; even though they were as powerful as the posterior extremities, they would suffer fracture or dislocation. We cannot but admire, therefore, the provision in all quadrupeds whose speed is great, and whose spring is extensive, that, from the structure of their bones, they have an elastic resistance, by which the shock of descending is diminished.

. If we observe the bones of the anterior extremity of the horse, we shall see that the scapula is oblique to the chest; the humerus, oblique to the scapula; and the bones of the fore arm at an angle with the humerus. Were these bones connected together in a straight line, end to end, the shock of alighting would be conveyed through a solid column, and the bones of the foot, or the joints, would suffer from the concussion. When the rider is thrown forwards on his hands, and more certainly when he is pitched on his shoulder, the collar bone is broken, because in man, this bone forms a link of connection between the shoulder and the trunk, so as to receive the whole shock; and the same would happen in the horse, the stag, and all quadrupeds of great strength and swiftness, were not the scapulæ sustained by muscles, and not by bone, and did not the bones recoil and fold up.

The horse-jockey runs his hand down the horse's neck, in a knowing way, and says, "this horse has got a heavy shoulder, he is a slow horse!" He is right, but he does not understand the matter; it is not possible that the shoulder can be too much loaded with muscle, for muscle is the source of motion, and bestows power. What the jockey feels, and forms his judgment on, is the abrupt transition from the neck to the shoulder, which, in a horse for the turf, ought to be a smooth undulating surface. This abruptness, or prominence of the shoulder, is a consequence of the upright position of the scapula; the sloping and light shoulder results from its obliquity. An upright shoulder is the mark of a stumbling horse : it does not revolve easily, to throw forward the foot.

Much of the strength, if not the freedom and rapidity of motion, of a limb, will depend on the angle at which the bones lie to each other ; for, this mainly affects the insertion, and, consequently, the power of the muscles. We know, and may every moment feel, that when the arm is extended, we possess little

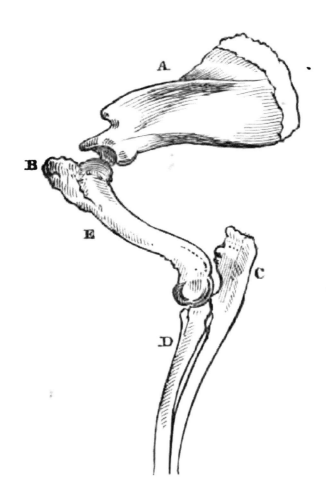

A. Scapula. E. Humerus. B. Tuberosity of the Humerus. C. Olecranon, or projection of the Ulna. D. Radius.

power in bending it ; but as we bend it the power is increased ; which is owing to the change in the direction of the force acting upon the bone ; or, in other words, because the tendon becomes more perpendicular to the lever. A scapula which inclines obliquely backwards, increases the angle at which it ies with the humerus, .and, consequently, improves the effect of those muscles which pass from it to the humerus. We have only to turn to the skeleton of the elephant, the ox, the elk, or the stag, to see the confirmation of this principle. When the scapula is oblique, the serratus muscle, which passes from the ribs to its uppermost part, has more power in rolling it. When it lies at right angles with the humerus, the muscles which are attached to the latter, (at B.) act with more effect. And on the same principle, by the oblique position of the humerus, and, consequently, its obliquity in reference to the radius and ulna, the power of the muscle inserted (at C.) into the olecranon, is increased. On the whole, both power and elasticity are gained by this position of the superior bones of the fore-leg. It gives to the animal that springs, a larger stretch in throwing himself forwards, and security, in a soft descent of his weight. A man, standing upright, cannot leap or start off at once ; he must first sink down, and bring the bones of his extremities to an angle. But the antelope, or other timid animals of the class, can leap at once, or start off in their course without preparation : another advantage of the oblique position of their bones when at rest.

The leg of the elephant is obviously built for the purpose of sustaining the huge bulk of the animal, whilst in the camel we have a perfect contrast.

Were we to compare the bones of these larger animals with any form of architecture, we might say, it was the Egyptian, or rather like the Cyclopean walls of some ancient city ; they are huge and shapeless, and piled over each other, as if they were

5*

destined more to sustain the weight, than to permit motion.

We further perceive, from the comparison of these sketches, that if the humerus be placed obliquely, it must necessarily be short, otherwise it would throw the leg too far back, and make the head and neck project. It is one of the " points" of a horse to have the humerus short. And not only have all animals of speed this character, but birds of long flight, as the swallow, have short humeri. This is owing, I think, to another circumstance, that in the wing, the short humerus causes a quicker extension; for the further extremity of the bone moving in a lesser circle, makes the gyration be more rapid.

If we take the bones of the shoulder as a distinct subject, and trace them comparatively, we shall be led to notice some very curious modifications in them. We have already seen that there are two objects to be attained in the construction of these bones. In man, and mammalia, they constitute an important part of the organ of respiration; and they conform to the structure of the thorax. But we shall find that in some animals, this function is in a manner withdrawn from them; the scapulæ and the clavicles are left without the support of the ribs.— These bones forming the shoulder, therefore, require additional carpentry; or they must be laid together on a new principle. In the batrachian order, for example in the frog, the thorax, as constituted of ribs, has disappeared; the mechanism of respiration is altogether different from what it is in the mammalia. Accordingly, we find that the bones of the shoulder are on a new model; they form a broad and flat circle, sufficient to give secure attachment to the extremity, and affording a large space for the lodgment of the muscles which move the arm.— Perhaps the best example of this structure is in the siren and proteus; where the ribs are reduced to a very few imperfect processes, attached to the anterior dorsal vertebræ; and where the bones of the extremity, being deprived of all support from the thorax, depend upon themselves for security. Here the bones, corresponding to the sternum, clavicles, and scapulæ, are found clinging to the spine, and forming, like the pelvis, a circle, to the lateral part of which the humerus is articulated.

In the chelonian order, the tortoises, we see another design accomplished, in the union of these bones; and the change is owing to a very curious circumstance. The spine and ribs of these animals form the rafters of their strong shell; and consequently they are external to the bones of the shoulder. The scapulæ and clavicles being thus within the thorax, and having nothing in their grasp, neither ribs nor spine, they must necessarily fall together, and form a circle, in order to afford a fixed point to which the extremity may be attached. It would, indeed, be

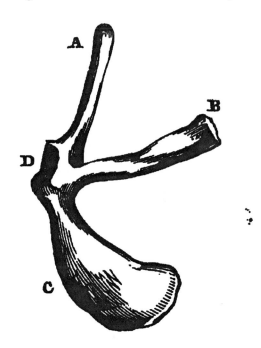

A. Scapula. B. Acromion process. c. Coracoid bone. D. Glenoid cavity.

strange if, now being joined for the purpose of giving attachment to the humerus, and in circumstances, as we may express it, so very new, they preserved any resemblance to the forms which we have been contemplating in the higher animals. In the figure on the preceding page, we have the bones of the shoulder of the turtle; and it is readily perceived how much they have changed both their shape and their offices. That part which is most like a scapula in shape, lies on the fore part, instead of the back part; and the bones which hold the shoulders apart, abut upon the spine, instead of upon the sternum. Hence it appears idle to follow out these bones under the old denominations, or such as are applicable to their condition in the higher animals.

In fishes, where the apparatus of respiration has undergone another entire change, and where there are no proper ribs, the bones which give attachment to the pectoral fin, are still called the bones of the shoulder; and that which is named scapular appendage, is, in fact, attached to the bones of the head. So that the whole consists of a circle of bones, which, we may say, seek security of attachment by approaching the more solid part of the head, in defect of a firm foundation in the thorax.

Thus, the bones which, in a manner, give a foundation to those of the anterior extremity, have been submitted to a new modelling, in correspondence with every variety in the apparatus of respiration; and they have yet maintained their pristine office.

The naturalist will not be surprised, on finding an extraordinary intricacy in the shoulder apparatus of the ornithorynchus paradoxus, since the whole frame and organs of this animal imply, that it is intermediate between mammalia and birds; and it is placed in the list of edentata. We introduce it here, as another instance of the changes which the bones of the shoulder undergo with every new office, and in correspondence with the motions, of the extremity;

whether it be to support the weight in running, or to give freedom to the arm, or to provide for flying, or

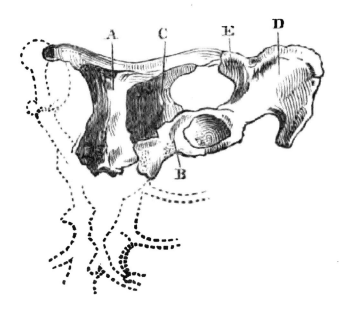

for performing equally the act of creeping and of swimming.

Unprofitable as the enquiry may seem, there is no other way by which the geologist can distinguish the genera of those oviparous reptiles, which he finds imbedded in the secondary strata, than by studying the minute processes and varying characters of these bones, in the different classes of animals. In the ichthyosaurus, and plesiosaurus, the inhabitants of a former world, and now extinct, we perceive a considerable deviation from the perfection of the bones of the arm and hand, compared with the frog and tortoise: but if strength is the object, there is a greater degree of perfection in the bones of the shoulder.   The explanation of this is, that the ribs and sterno-costal arches, constituting the thorax are more perfect, than in

A. Clavicle. B. Coracoid bone. c. A new bone, introduced into the apparatus, which articulates with the coracoid bone, and lies interior to the clavicle. D. Scapula. E. Acromion Scapulæ.

the chelonian and batrachian orders; and the bones
of the shoulder are therefore external, and resemble
those of the crocodile; yet the ribs are so weak as to
be incapable of sustaining the powerful action of the
anterior extremities; accordingly, the bones, which
by a kind of licence we continue to call clavicle,
omoplate or scapula, and coracoid, though strangely
deviating from the original form and connections,
constitute a texture of considerable strength, which
perfects the anterior part of the trunk, and gives
attachment and lodgment to the powerful muscles of
the paddle.

But in giving their attention to this subject, it does
not appear that naturalists have hit upon the right
explanation of the peculiar structure, and curious
varieties of these bones. Why is the apparatus of
respiration so totally changed in these classes of animals? They are cold blooded animals; they require
to respire less frequently than other creatures, and
they remain long under water. I conceive that the
peculiarity in their mode of respiration corresponds
with this property. Hence their vesicular lungs,
their mode of swallowing the air, instead of inhaling
it; and hence, especially, their power of compressing
the body and expelling the air; it is this, I imagine,
which enables them to go under the water and crawl
upon the bottom; without this, that is to say, had they
possessed the lungs of warm blooded animals, which
are compressible only in a slight degree, their capacity of remaining under water would have left them
struggling against their buoyancy, like a man or
any of the mammalia when diving. The girdle of
bones of the shoulder is constituted with a certain
regard to the peculiar action of respiration, and to
the pliancy of the body, in order that the vesicular
lungs may be compressed, and the specific weight
diminished. The facility which the absence of ribs
gives, in the batrachian order, and the extreme
weakness and pliancy of these bones in the saurians,

for admitting the compression of the lungs extended through the abdomen, must be, as I apprehend, peculiarities adapted to the same end.

OF THE HUMERUS.

The demonstration of this bone need not be so dry a matter of detail as the anatomist makes it. We may see in it that curious relation of parts which has been so successfully employed by Paley to prove design, and from which the genius of Baron Cuvier has brought out some of the finest examples of inductive reasoning.

In looking to the head of this bone in the human skeleton, (see the fig. page 43,) we observe the great hemispherical surface for articulation with the glenoid cavity of the scapula, and we see that the two tubercles, near the joint, are depressed, and do not interfere with the revolving of the humerus, by striking against the scapula.

Such appearances alone are sufficient to show that all the motions of the arm are free. To give assurance of this, suppose that the geologist has picked up this bone in interesting circumstances. To what animal does it belong? The circular form of the articulating surface, and the very slight projection of the tubercles, evince a latitude and extent of motion. Now, freedom of motion in the shoulder, implies freedom also in the extremity or paw, and rotation of the bones of the wrist. Accordingly, we direct the eye to that part of this humerus which gives origin to the muscles for turning the wrist, (the *Supinator muscles*), and in the prominence and length of the ridge or crest which is on the lower and outer side of the bone, we have proof of the free motion of the paw.

Therefore, on finding the humerus thus characterized, we conclude, that it belonged to an animal with sharp moveable claws ; that, in all probability, it is the remains of a bear.

But, suppose that the bone found has a different character :—That the tubercles project, so as to limit the motion to one direction, and that the articulating surface is less regularly convex. On inspecting the lower extremity of such a bone, we shall perceive provisions for a deeper and more secure hinge-joint at the elbow ; and neither in the form of the articulating surface, (which is here called trochlea), nor in the spine on the outside, above noticed, will there be signs of the rotation of one bone of the fore arm on the other. We have, therefore, got the bone of an herbivorous quadruped, either with a solid or with a cloven foot.

In the bat and mole we have, perhaps, the best examples of the moulding of the bones of the extremity, to correspond with the condition of the animal. The mole is an animal fitted to plough its way under ground. In the bat, the same system of bones is adapted to form a wing, to raise the animal in the atmosphere ; and with a provision to cling to the wall, not to bear upon. We recognize in both, every bone of the upper extremity, but how very differently formed and joined ! In the mole, the sternum or breast bone, and the clavicle are remarkably large : the scapula assumes the form of a high lever : the humerus is thick and short, and has such spines for the attachment of muscles, as indicate great power. The spines, which give origin to the muscles of rotation, project in an extraordinary manner ; and the hand is large, flat, and so turned, that it may shove the earth aside like a ploughshare.*

* The snout may vary in its internal structure with new offices. Naturalists say that there is a new " element" in the pig's nose. It has, in fact, two bones which admit of motion, whilst they give more strength. Moles have those bones also, as they plough the earth with their snouts. We have noticed the manner in which they use their strong hands ; we should add that their head is a wedge, to

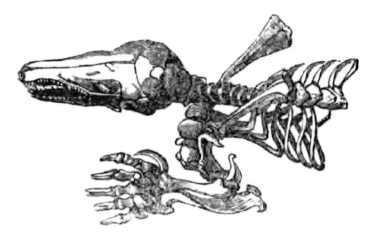

There can be no greater contrast to these bones than is presented in the skeleton of the bat. In

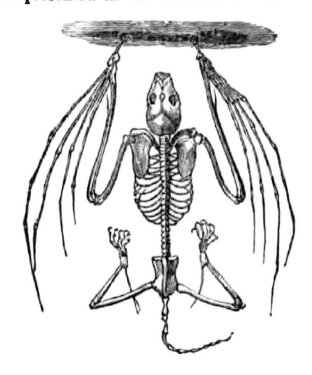

which their hands are assisting, in throwing aside the earth. The conformation of the head in shape and strength of bones, and the new adjustment of a muscle, which is cutaneous in other animals (the *Platisma Myoides*) to the motions of the head, are among the most curious changes of common parts to new offices.

that animal the bones are light and delicate; and whilst they are all marvellously extended, the phalanges of the fingers are elongated, so as hardly to be recognized, obviously for the purpose of sustaining a membraneous web, and to form a wing.

Contemplating this extraordinary application of the bones of the extremity, and comparing them with those in the wing of a bird, we might say, that this is an awkward attempt—a failure. But before giving expression to such an opinion, we must understand the objects required in this construction.— It is not a wing intended merely for flight, but one which, while it raises the animal, is capable of receiving a new sensation, or sensations in that exquisite degree, so as almost to constitute a new sense. On the fine web of the bat's wing, nerves are distributed, which enable it to avoid objects in its flight, during the obscurity of night, when both eyes and ears fail. Could the wing of a bird, covered with feathers, do this? Here then we have another example of the necessity of taking every circumstance into consideration before we presume to criticise the ways of nature. It is a lesson of humility.*

In the next page we have a sketch of the arm bones of the Ant-eater,† to shew once more the correspondence in the whole extremity. We observe these extraordinary spines of the humerus marking the power of the muscles which are attached to it; for as I have said before, whether we examine the human body, or the comparative forms of the bones, the distinctness of the spines and processes declares the strength of the muscles. It is particularly pleas-

* Besides the adaptation of the bat for flight, through a new adjustment of the bones of the arm, this animal has cells under its skin; but I know not how far I am authorized to say that they are analogous to the air-cells of birds, or that they are for the purpose of making the bat specifically lighter. They extend over the breast, and under the axillæ in some bats; and they are filled by an orifice which communicates with the pharynx.

† Tamandua, from South America.

ing to notice here the correspondence between the humerus and the other bones, the scapula large and with a double spine, and with great processes: the ulna projecting at the olecranon, and the radius freely rotating: but above all, in the developement of one grand metacarpal bone, which gives attachment to a strong claw, we see a very distinct provision for scratching and turning aside the ant-hill. The whole

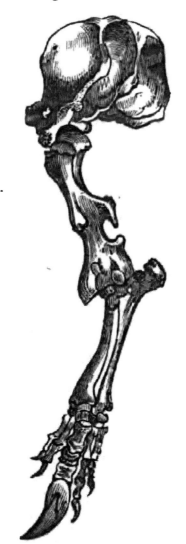

is an example of the relation of the particular parts
of the skeleton to one another; and were it our busi-
ness, it would be easy to shew, that as there is a correspondence among the bones of the arm, so is there
a more universal relation between those of the whole
skeleton.   As the structure of the bones declares the
provision of the extremity for digging into the ant-
hills, so we shall not be disappointed in our expectation of finding a projecting muzzle unarmed with
teeth, and a long tongue provided with a glutinous
secretion, to lick up the emmets which are disturbed
by the animal's scratching.

In the skeleton of the cape-mole, we may see, from
the projecting acromion scapulæ, and a remarkable
process of the humerus, that there is a provision for
the rotation of the arm, which implies burrowing.
But the apparatus seems by no means so perfect as in
the mole, implying that it digs in a softer soil than
that animal, whilst the possession of gnawing teeth
indicates that it lives on roots.

In BIRDS there is altogether a new condition of
parts, as there is a new element to contend with.
The very peculiar form and structure of their skeleton may be thus accounted for.   First, it is necessary
that birds, as they are buoyed in the air, be specifically lighter.   Secondly, the circumference of their
thorax must be extended, and the motions of their
ribs limited, that the muscles of the wings may have
sufficient space and firmness for their attachment.
Both these objects are attained by a modification of
the apparatus of breathing.   The lungs are highly
vascular and spongy, but they are not distended with
air.   The air is drawn through their substance into
the large cavity common to the chest and abdomen;
and whilst the great office of decarbonization of the
blood is securely performed, advantage is taken to let
the air into all the cavities, even into those of the
bones.   From what was said in the introductory
chapter, of the weight of the body being a necessary

concomitant of muscular strength, we see why birds, by reason of their lightness, as well as by the conformation of their skeleton, walk badly. And, on the other hand, in observing how this lightness is adapted for flight, it is remarkable how small an addition to their body will prevent them rising on the wing. If the griffon-vulture be frightened after his repast, he must disgorge, before he flies ; and the condor, in the same circumstances, is taken by the Indians, like a quadruped, by throwing the lasso over it.*

As every one must have observed, the breast-bone of birds extends the whole length of the body ; and owing to this extension, a lesser degree of motion suffices to respiration. So that a greater surface, necessary for the lodgement and attachment of the muscles of the wings, is obtained, whilst that surface is less disturbed by the action of breathing, and is more steady. Another peculiarity of the skeleton of the bird is the consolidation of the vertebræ of the back ; a proof, if any were now necessary, that the whole system of bones conforms to that of the extremities, the firmer texture of the bones of the trunk, being a part of the provision for the attachment of the muscles of the wings.†

The vertebræ of the back being fixed in birds, and the pelvis reaching high, there is no motion in the body ; indeed, if there were, it would be interrupted by the sternum. We cannot but admire, therefore, the composition of the neck and head, and how the extension of the vertebræ, and the length and pliability of the neck, whilst they give to the bill the office of a hand, become a substitution for the loss of

---

* It is interesting to notice the relations of great functions in the animal economy. Birds are oviparous, because they never could have risen on the wing had they been viviparous ; if the full stomach of a carnivorous bird retard its flight, we perceive that it could not have carried its young. The light body, the quill-feathers, the bill, and the laying of eggs, are all necessarily connected.

† The ostrich and cassowary, which are rather runners than fliers, have the spine loose.

motion in the body, by balancing the whole, as in standing, running, or flying. Is it not curious to observe how the whole skeleton is adapted to this one object, the power of the wings.

Whilst the ostrich has no keel in its breast-bone, birds of passage are, on dissection, recognisable by the depth of this ridge of the sternum. The reason is that the angle, formed by this process and the body of the bone, affords lodgement for the pectoral muscle, the powerful muscle of the wing. In this sketch of the dissection of the swallow, there is a curious resemblance to the human arm, and we cannot fail to observe, that the pectoral muscle constitutes the greater part of the bulk of the body.* And here we see the correspondence between the strength of this muscle and the rate of flying of the swallow, which is a mile in a minute, for ten hours every day, or six hundred miles a day.† If it be true that birds, when migrating, require a wind that blows against them, it implies an extraordinary power, as well as continuance of muscular exertion.

We see how Nature completes her work, when the intention is that the animal shall rise buoyant and powerful in the air :—the whole texture of the frame is altered and made light, in a manner consistent with strength. We see also how the mechanism of the anterior extremity is changed, and the muscles of the trunk differently directed. But we are tempted to examine those means, which we would almost say are more awkwardly suited for their purpose, where the system of bones and muscles, peculiar to the quadruped, is preserved, while a power of launching into the air is also given. We have already

---

* Borelli makes the pectoral muscles of a bird, exceed in weight all the other muscles taken together; whilst the pectoral muscles of man, are but a seventieth part of the whole mass of the muscles.

† Mr. White ~ys truly, that the swift lives on the wing; it eats, drinks, and collects materials for its nest in flying, and never rests but during darkness.

noticed the structure of the bat as adapted to flight; but there are other animals which enjoy this function in a lesser degree. For example, the flying squirrel (Petromys Volucella), being chased to the end of the bough, spreads out its mantle from one extremity to the other, and drops in the air; but with such a resistance from its extended skin and its tail, that it can direct its flight obliquely downwards, and even turn in the air. But to this end, there is no necessity for any adaptation of the anterior extremity. Among reptiles there is a provision of the same kind, in the Draco fimbriatus; which is capable of creeping to a height, and dropping safely to the ground, under the protection of a sort of parachute, formed by its extended skin. This is not an inapt illustration, for although the phalanges of the fingers are not here used to extend the web, the ribs, which are unnecessary for breathing, are prolonged like the whalebone of an umbrella, and on them the skin is expanded.

But this brings us to a very curious subject,—the condition of those Saurian reptiles, the remains of which are found only in a fossil state, in what are termed the ancient strata of the Jura. The Pterodactyle of Cuvier is an animal which seems to confound all our notions of system. Its mouth was like the long bill of a bird, and its flexible neck corresponded; but it had teeth in its jaws like those of a crocodile. It had the bones of the anterior extremity prolonged, and fashioned somewhat like those in the wing of a bird; but it could not have had feathers, as it had not a proper bill. We see no creature having feathers without a bill to dress and prim them. Nor did this extremity resemble the structure in that of a bat: instead of the phalanges being equally prolonged, the second only was extended to an extraordinary length, whilst the third, fourth, and fifth remained with the length and articulation of a quadruped, and with sharp nails, corresponding with the pointed teeth. The extended metacarpal bone reached double the whole length of the animal, and the conjecture is, that upon it was extended a membrane, resembling that of the Draco fimbriatus. In the imperfect specimens which we have, we cannot discover in the height of the pelvis, the strength of the vertebræ of the back, or the expansion of the sternum, a provision for the attachment of muscles commensurate with the extent of the supposed wing. The humerus, and the bones, which we presume are the scapula and coracoid, bear some correspondence to the extent of the wing ; but the extraordinary circumstance of all, is the size and strength of the bones of the jaw and vertebræ of the neck, compared with the smallness of the body, and the extreme delicacy of the ribs ; which make it, altogether, the thing most incomprehensible in nature.

OF THE RADIUS AND ULNA.

The easy motion of the hand, we might imagine to be in the hand itself ; but, on the contrary, the movements which appear to belong to it, are divided among all the bones of the extremity.*

The head of the humerus is rotatory on the scapula, as when making the guards in fencing ; but the easier and finer rolling of the wrist is accomplished by the motion of the radius on the ulna.

The ulna has a hooked process, the olecranon, which catches round the lower end of the humerus or arm bone, (this articulating portion is called trochlea), and forms with it a hinge joint. The radius, again, has a small, neat, round head, which is bound to the ulna by ligaments, as a spindle is held in the bush. This bone turns on its axis and, as it turns,

---

* In the sketch in the next page, the upper bone of the fore-arm is the radius, and in revolving on the lower bone, the ulna, it carries the hand with it.

carries the hand with it, because the hand is strictly attached to its lower head alone. This rolling, is what is termed pronation and supination.

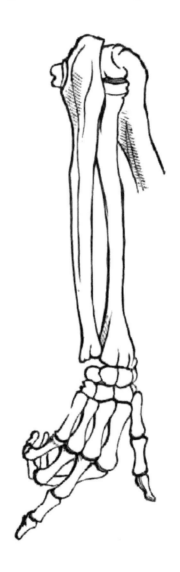

Such a motion would be useless, and a source of weakness in an animal that had a solid hoof. Accordingly, in the horse, these bones are united together and consolidated in the positon of pronation.

It is interesting to find that by studying the processes of the bones, than which nothing, at first sight, appears more inconsequent, we are learning the characters of a language which shall enable us to read monuments of the highest interest ;—the records of the creation, which give an account of the revolutions of the earth itself.

If a geologist should find the nearer head of the radius, and see in the extremity of it a smooth depression, where it bears against the humerus, and observe the polished circle that turns on the cavity of the ulna,—he would say,—This animal had a paw—it had a motion at the wrist, which implies claws. Claws may belong to two species of animals : the feline, which is possessed of sharp carnivorous teeth, or to animals without teeth. If he should find the lower extremity of this same bone, and observe on it spines and grooves for the distinct tendons which disperse to the phalanges, he would conclude that there must have been moveable claws—that it belonged to a carnivorous animal ; and he would seek for canine teeth of a corresponding size.

OF THE WRIST AND HAND.

In the human hand, the bones of the wrist (carpus) are eight in number ; and they are so closely connected that they form a sort of ball, which moves on the end of the radius. Beyond these, and towards the fingers are the metacarpal bones, which diverge at their further extremities, and give support to the bones of the fingers. The thumb has no metacarpal bone, and is directly articulated with the carpus or wrist. There are thus in the hand twenty-nine bones, from the mechanism of which, result strength, mobility, and elasticity.

Lovers of system (I do not use the term disparagingly) delight to trace the gradual substraction of the bones of the hand. Thus, looking to the hand of man, they see the thumb fully formed—in the simiæ they find it exceedingly small; in one of them, the spider-monkey, it has disappeared, and the four fingers are sufficient, with hardly the rudiments of a thumb. In some of the tardigrade animals, there are only three metacarpal bones with their fingers. In the horse, the cannon bone may be shewn to consist of two metacarpal bones. Indeed, we might go further and instance the wing of the bird. To me, this appears to be losing the sense, in the love of system. There is no regular gradation, but a variety, most curiously adapting, as I have often to repeat, the same system of parts to every necessary purpose.

In a comparative view of these bones, we are led more particularly to notice the foot of the horse; it is universally admitted to be of a beautiful design, and calculated for strength and elasticity, and especially provided against concussion.

The bones of the fore-leg of the horse become firmer as we trace them downwards. The two bones corresponding with those of the fore-arm, are braced together and consolidated; and the motion at the elbow joint is limited to flexion and extension. The carpus, forming what by a sort of license is called the knee, is also new modelled; but the metacarpal bones and phalanges of the toes are totally changed, and can hardly be recognized. When we look in front, instead of the four metacarpal bones, we see one strong bone, the cannon bone, and posterior to this, we find two lesser bones, called splint bones. The heads of these lesser bones enter into the knee-joint; but at their lower ends they diminish gradually, and they are held by an elastic ligamentous attachment to the sides of the cannon bone.

I have some hesitation in admitting the correctness of the opinion of veterinary surgeons of this curious piece of mechanism. They imagine that these moveable splint bones, by playing up and down, as the foot is alternately raised and pressed to the ground, bestow elasticity and prevent concussion.— The fact certainly is, that by over action this part becomes inflamed, and the extremities are preternaturally joined by bone to the greater metacarpal or cannon bone; and that this, which is called a splint, is a cause of lameness.

I suspect, rather, that in the perfect state of the joint, these lesser metacarpal bones act as a spring to throw out the foot, when it is raised and the knee-joint bent. If we admit that it is the quickness in the extension of this joint on which the rate of motion must principally depend, it will not escape observation, that in the bent position of the knee, the extensor tendons have very little power, owing to their

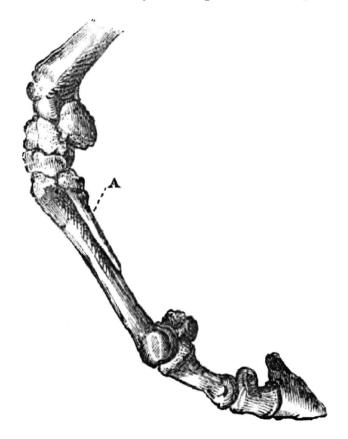

running so near the centre of motion in the joint; and that, in fact, they require some additional means to aid the extension of the leg.

Suppose that the head of the lesser metacarpal bone A enters into the composition of the joint, it does not appear that by its yielding, when the foot is upon the ground, the bones of the carpus can descend, as long as they are sustained by the greater metacarpal or cannon bone. I do not, therefore, conceive that this bone can add to the elasticity of the foot. But when we perceive that the head of the splint bone is behind the centre of motion in the joint, it is obvious that it must be more pressed upon, in the bent condition of the joint when the foot is elevated, and that then, the bone must descend. If it be depressed when the foot is raised, and have a power of recoiling (which it certainly has) it must aid in throwing out the leg into the straight position and assist the extensor muscles. Further, we can readily believe that when the elasticity of these splint bones is lost, by ossification uniting them firmly to the cannon bone, the want of such a piece of mechanism, essential to the quick extension of the foot, will make the horse apt to come down.

In looking to this sketch, and comparing it with that of the hand on page 69, we see that in the horse's leg the five bones of the first digital phalanx are consolidated into the large pastern bone; those of the second phalanx, into the lesser pastern or coronet; and those of the last phalanx, into the coffin bone.

OF THE HORSE'S FOOT.—But the foot itself deserves our attention. The horse, a native of extensive plains and steppes, is perfect in his structure, as adapted to these, his natural pasture grounds. When brought, however, into subjection, and running on our hard roads, his feet suffer from concussion. The value of the horse, so often impaired by lameness of the foot, has made that part an object of great interest : and I have it from the excellent professor of veterinary surgery to say, that he has never demonstrated the anatomy of the horse's foot without finding something new to admire.

The weight and power of the animal require that he should have a foot in which strength and elasticity are combined. The elasticity is essentially necessary to prevent percussion in striking the ground ; and it is attained here, through the united effect of the oblique position of the bones of the leg and foot —the yielding nature of the suspending ligament, and the expansibility of the crust or hoof. So much depends on the position of the pastern bones and coffin bone, that judging by the length of these and their obliquity, it is possible to say whether a horse goes easily, without mounting it. When the hoof is raised, it is smaller in its diameter, and the sole is concave ; but when it bears on the ground it expands, the sole descends so as to become flatter ; and this expansion of the hoof laterally, is necessary to the play of the whole structure of the foot. Hence it happens that if the shoe be nailed in such a manner as to prevent the hoof expanding, the whole interior contrivance for mobility and elasticity is lost. The foot, in trotting, comes down solid, it consequently suffers percussion ; and from the injury, it becomes inflamed and hot. From this inflammation is generated a variety of diseases, which at length destroy all the beautiful provision of the horse's foot for free and elastic motion.

This subject is of such general interest, that I may venture on a little more detail. The elastic or suspending ligament spoken of above, passes down from the back of the cannon bone, along all the bones, to the lowest, the coffin bone ; it yields, and allows these bones to bend. Behind the ligament the great tendons run, and the most prolonged of these, that of the perforans muscle, is principally inserted into the coffin bone, having at the same time

other attachments.   Under the bones and tendon, at
the sole of the foot, there is a soft elastic cushion ;
this cushion rests on the proper horny frog, that
prominence of a triangular shape which is seen in
the hollow of the sole. · The soft elastic matter being
pressed down, shifts a little backwards, so that it
expands the heels at the same time that it bears on
the frog, and presses out the lateral part of the crust.
We perceive that there is a necessity for the bottom
of the hoof being hollow or concave—first, to prevent
the delicate apparatus of the foot from being bruised,
and, secondly, that elasticity may be obtained by its
descent.   We see that the expansion of the hoof, and
the descent of the sole are necessary to the play of
the internal apparatus of the foot.

That there is a relation between the internal structure and the covering, whether it be the nail, or crust,
or hoof, we can hardly doubt : and an unexpected
proof of this offers itself in the horse.   There are
some very rare instances of a horse having digital extremities.   According to Suetonius, there was
such an animal in the stables of Cæsar ; another
was in the possession of Leo X.; and Geoffrey St.
Hilaire, in addition to those, says, that he has seen a
horse with three toes on the fore-foot, and four on
the hind-foot.*   These instances of deviation in the
natural structure of the bones were accompanied
with a corresponding change in the coverings—the
toes had nails, not hoofs.

By these-examples, it is made to appear still more
distinctly that there is a relation between the internal configuration of the toes and their coverings—
that when there are five toes complete in their bones,
they are provided with perfect nails—when two toes
represent the whole, as in the cleft foot of the rumin-

* Such a horse was not long since exhibited in Town and at
Newmarket.

ant, there are appropriate horny coverings—and that when the bones are joined to form the pastern bones and coffin bone, there is a hoof or crust, as in the horse, couagga, zebra, and ass.

In ruminants there is a cannon bone, but the foot is split into two parts, and this must add to its spring or elasticity. I am inclined to think that there is still another intention in this form; it prevents the foot sinking in soft ground, and permits it to be more easily withdrawn. We may observe how much more easily the cow withdraws her foot from the yielding margin of a river, than the horse. The round and concave form of the horse's foot is attended with a vacuum or suction, as it is withdrawn; while the split and conical shaped hoof expands in sinking, and is easily extricated.

In the chamois and other species of the deer there is an additional toe. A sort of lesser cannon bone, with its two pasterns, supports this toe, and is joined by ligament to the larger cannon bone, so that it must have great elasticity. As a division of the flexor tendon runs into it, it must increase the spring when the animal rises from its crouching position. We see, in these sketches, that the lesser metacarpal bone, which, in the horse, entered into the joint of the "knee," is here brought down to increase the elasticity, or to expand the foot.

The two lateral toes of the hog are short, and do not touch the ground, yet they must serve to sustain the animal when the foot sinks. In the rein-deer these bones are strong and deep, and the toe, by projecting backwards, extends the foot horizontally—thus giving the animal a broader base to stand on, and adapting it to the snows of Lapland, on the principle of the snow-shoe. The systematic naturalist will call these changes in the size, number, and place of the metacarpal bones " gradations;" I see in them only new proofs of the same system of bones being applicable to every circumstance, or condition of animals, and furnishing us with other instances of *adaptation*.

I have explained why I think that the bones of the elephant's leg stand so perpendicularly over each other; there is a peculiarity also in the bones of the foot. In the foot of the living animal we see only a round pliant mass, which, when he stands, resembles the base of a pillar, or the lower part of the trunk of a stately tree. But when we examine the bones of the foot, we find this broad base to consist of the carpus, metacarpus, and phalanges of the toes; and these bones have a very different use from what we have hitherto noticed. They are not connected with a moveable radius, and have no individual motion, as in the carnivorous animal—they merely serve to expand the foot, the base of the column, and to give it a certain elasticity.

In page 53 I have noticed the bones of the foot of the camel in contrast with those of the elephant. The camel's foot having no such disproportioned weight to bear as in the elephant, lightness of motion is secured by the oblique position of its bones, as well as by the direction of the bones of the shoulder, which we have formerly noticed. In the soft texture of the camel's foot there is much to admire; for although the bottom be flat, like the sole of a shoe, yet there is between it and the bones and tendons a cushion, so soft and elastic that the animal treads with great lightness and security. The resemblance of the foot of the ostrich to that of the camel has not escaped naturalists.

We are now treating of the last bones of the toes; and let us see what may be done, by the study of one of these bones, to the bodying forth of the whole animal. I allude to the dissertations of the President Jefferson and Baron Cuvier on the Megalonix. But we must preface this part of our subject by some remarks on the form of the claws of the lion.

The canine tribe are carnivorous, like the feline,

7*

and both have the last bones of their toes armed with a nail or claw. But their habits and their means of obtaining food are different. The first combine a keen sense of smelling with a power of continued speed; they run down their prey. The feline order have their superiority in the fineness of their sight, accompanied with a patience, watchfulness, and stealthy movement; they spring upon their prey, and never long pursue it. They attain their object in a few bounds, and, failing, sulkily resume their watch. When we look to the claws, we see a correspondence with those habits. The claws of the dog and wolf are coarse and strong, and bear the pressure and friction incident to a long chase. They are calculated to sustain and protect the foot. But the tiger leaps on his prey, and fastens his sharp and crooked claws in the flesh. These claws being curved and sharp, we must admire the mechanism by which they are preserved. The last bone, that which supports the claw, is placed lateral to the penultimate bone, and is so articulated with it, that an elastic ligament (A) draws it back and raises the sharp extremity of the claw upwards. The nearer extremity of the furthest bone presses the ground in the ordinary running of the animal,* whilst the

* The pads in the bottom of the lion's foot cover these bones, or rather, we should say, protect them; they are soft cushions, which add to the elasticity of the foot, and must, in some degree, defend the animal in alighting from its bound. I could not comprehend how the powerful flexor muscles did not unsheath the claws when the lion made its spring, and how they produced this effect when there was an excitement to seize and hold the prey—I made this dissection to detect the cause. The last bone of the toe is placed in a manner so peculiar in relation to the penultimate, being drawn back by the elastic ligament (A) beyond the centre of motion of the joint, that the flexor tendon (B) acting upon it, forces the nearer end, and the cushion of the toe to the ground. But when a more general excitement takes place in the muscles called interossei, and the extensors, D, E, the relative position of the two last bones is altered; so that the action of the flexor tendon can now draw forward the last bone—thus unsheathing and uncovering the claw, and preparing it to hold or to tear.

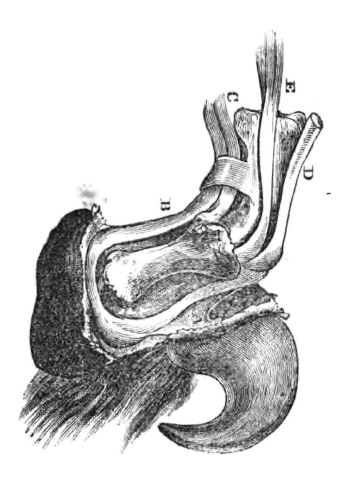

claw is thus retracted into a sheath. Bv
tiger makes his spring, the claws are v
action of the flexor tendons ; and th
and strong in the Bengal tiger, r
powerful, that they have been k
man's skull by a touch, in th
him.

I have alluded to the ob
ferson on the Megaloni
which by its articulati
he recognised to be c
of an animal of greal
cover that it had carrieo

cumstance, he naturally enough concluded (according to the adage—ex ungue leonem) that it must have belonged to a carnivorous animal. He next set about calculating the length of this claw, and estimating the size of the animal. He satisfied himself that in this bone, a relic of the ancient world, he had obtained a proof of the existence, during these old times, of a lion of the height of the largest ox, and an opponent fit to cope with the mastodon. But when this bone came under the scrutiny of Baron Cuvier, his perfect knowledge of anatomy enabled him to draw a different conclusion.

He first observed that there was a spine in the middle of the articulating surface of the last bone, which in this respect was unlike the form of the same bone in the feline tribe. He found no provision in this specimen of an extinct animal, for the lateral attachment of the bone, which we have just noticed to be necessary for its retraction. Then observing what portion of a circle this bone formed, he prolonged the line, and showed that the claw belonging to it must have been of such great length, that it could never have been retracted to the effect of guarding an acute and sharp point. The point, therefore, could not have been raised vertically, so as to have permitted the animal to put the foot to the ground without blunting the instrument! Pursuing such a comparison, he rejected the idea of the bone belonging to the feline tribe at all. His attention was directed to another order, the paresseux or sloths, which have great toes and long nails. Their nails are folded up in a different fashion; they just enable the animal to walk; but slowly and awkwardly, something in the same manner as if we were to fold our fingers on the palm of the hand, and bear upon our knuckles. On instituting a more just comparison between these bones of the ancient animal, and the corresponding bones of the paresseux, he has satisfied us, that the lion of the American President

was an animal which scratched the ground and fed
on roots.

One experiences something like relief to find that
there never was such an enormous carnivorous animal as this, denominated megalonix.

These finger-bones, or bones of the claws, exhibit
a very remarkable correspondence with the habits
and general forms of animals. Besides what we
have seen in the lion, or tiger, in the dog, and wolf,
in the bear ·and ant-eater, there is a variety, where
we should least expect it, in the animals that live in
woods, and climb the branches of trees. The squirrel, with claws set both ways, runs with equal facility
up and down the bole, and nestles in the angles of
the branches. The monkey leaps and swings himself from branch to branch, and springing, parts with
his hold by the hinder extremities before he reaches
with the anterior extremities ; he leaps the interven-
ing space, and catches with singular precision. But
the sloths do not grasp ; their fingers are like hooks,
and their strength is in their arms. They do not
hold, but hang to the branch. They never let
go with one set of hooks, until they have caught
with the other, and thus they use both hind and
fore feet, whilst their bodies are pendant. Here,
once more, we see the form of the extremity, the
concentration of strength, and the habit of animals, conforming not merely to their haunts in the
forest, but to their mode of moving and living among
the branches; all active, but in a different manner.

There have been of late deposited in our Museum
in the College of Surgeons, the bones of an animal of
great size; and the examination of these gives us an
opportunity of applying the principles and the mode of
investigation followed by our great authority in this
part of science.

These remains consist of part of the head, spine,
tail, pelvis, and the bones of one hinder extremity,
and the scapula. Estimating the animal at seven

feet in height, it scarcely conveys an adequate idea
of its size; for the thigh-bone is three times the diameter of that of the large elephant which is in the
same collection, and the pelvis is twice the breadth
of that of the same animal. Forming our opinion
on these principles to which we have had repeated
occasion to refer in this essay, and judging by the
strength and prominence of the processes of these
bones, the animal must have possessed great muscular power; and directed by the same circumstances
still, we can form an idea of the manner in which
that muscular power was employed.

On comparing these bones with the drawings of
the skeleton of the enormous animal preserved in the
Royal Museum of Madrid, it is seen at once that this
new acquisition is part of the remains of the great
animal of Paraguay, the Megatherium of Cuvier.
Every observation which we are enabled to make on
the extreme bones of the foot, on the scapula, and on
the teeth, confirms the idea entertained by Cuvier, that
it was a vegetable feeder; and that its great strength
was employed in flinging up the soil and digging for
roots. Its strength seems to have been concentrated to its paws, corresponding with the provisions
there for enormous nails or claws. I have heard it
surmised that this animal may have sat upon its
hinder extremities, and pulled down the branches of
trees to feed upon. It is only its great size that can
countenance such an idea. We have not the humerus, which by its processes would have declared
the classification and activity of its muscles; but we
can estimate the height, breadth, and strength of the
animal by the pelvis and enormous bones of the posterior extremity; while by the scapula and clavicle
we can form a conception of the extent of motion of
the anterior extremity, and the great power that it
possessed. In short, by the osseous and muscular
systems we perceive that the strength was not so
much in the body, certainly not in the jaws, but was

directed rather to the extremities; and that it was given neither for rapidity of motion nor defence, but for digging.

How little was it to be expected that an alliance between anatomy, the most despised part of it, and mineralogy, was to give rise to a new science;—making a part of natural history which had been pursued in mere idleness, vaguely, and somewhat fancifully, to be henceforth studied philosophically, and by inductive reasoning. It is both interesting and in-instructive to find the relations thus established between departments of knowledge apparently so remote. .

In the true Amphibia, as the phoca and walrus, we have the feet contracted, and almost enveloped in the skin, and the fingers webbed and converted into fins.

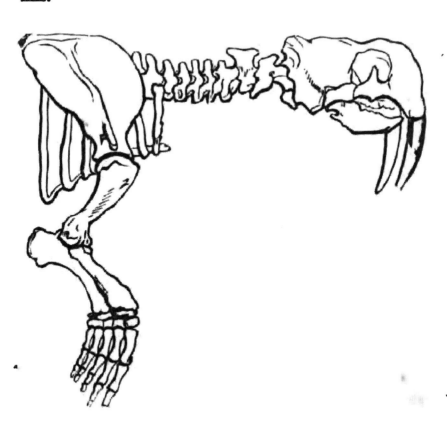

We have sketched here, the bones of the morse, or walrus, and they are remarkably complete, if we consider the appearance of the feet in the living animal. The bones are here accommodated to an instrument for swimming; for these animals live in the water, and come to land only to suckle their young, or to bask in the sun; and they are the most unwieldy and helpless, out of the water, of all animals which breathe.

In the Cetacea, we have mammalia without hind feet. The scapula is large, the humerus very short, and the bones of the fore-arm and hand flattened and confined in membranes which convert them into a fin. They live in the water, but must rise to breathe.

I need not say that in the dolphin we recognize the bones of the anterior extremity, only a little further removed from the forms which we have hitherto been contemplating. The seal and morse raise themselves out of the water and lie on the rocks; the different species of the dolphin continue always in the the water; the extremity is now a fin or an oar, and those who have seen the porpoise or the pelloch in a stormy sea, must acknowledge how complete the apparatus is, through which they enjoy their element.

The last examples I select, shall be from the ancient world.*

---

* The figure to the left is the anterior extremity of the Plesiosaurus; to the right that of the Ichthyosaurus. In these paddles we see the intermediate changes from the foot of land animals to the fin of the fish.—The walrus, dolphin, turtle, plesiosaurus, ichthyosaurus —where we no longer find the phalanges or attempt to count the bones. They become irregular polygons or trapezoids—less like the phalanges than the radii of the fins of a fish. In fishes the anterior extremity is recognized in the thoracic fin; and we may even discover the prototypes of the scapula and the bones of the arm. I know not what the naturalist, who likes to note the gradual decrease of the elementary parts, makes of these hundred bones of the paddle or of the fin; where there is an increase of the number, whilst, relatively speaking, there is a defect of form and motion, of the parts.

These figures are taken from specimens in the College of Surgeons, of fossil animals of singular structure, between the crocodile and the fish. They are in a calcareous rock, and the skeletons are entire, but crushed, and a good deal disfigured. Here are the

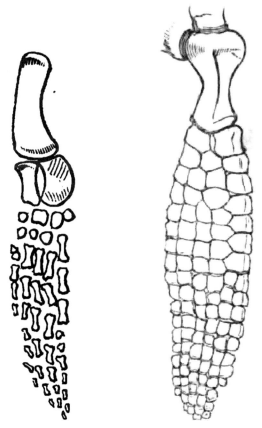

extremities or paddles consisting of a multitude of bones articulated ; and among these we still discover the humerus, radius and ulna, and bones of the carpus and fingers. No fault is to be found with the construction of these instruments ; they are suited to their offices, and no bone is superfluous, or misplaced, or imperfect. The ichthyosaurus and plesiosaurus (the animals which offer these specimens) inhabited the sea ; the remains are found low in the lias deposit ; great changes have been wrought on the land

and on the deep since they existed ; and the race of animals, the structure of whose extremities we have been engaged in examining, were not then in being. When we discover the same series of bones in the animals of the old world, we admit the existence of the same system ; and we must necessarily acknowledge the progressive developement of that system, through a period of time incalculably remote ; even if, instead of our days and years, referable to history, each day were as a thousand years, or we were to make our estimate by the records of the revolutions which have left their traces on the globe itself.

I have now given, I hope, sufficient examples of the changes in the bones of the anterior extremity, which suit them to every possible variety of use. After a little attention to the form of the human hand, I shall take up another division of my subject. The motions of the fingers do not merely result from the action of the large muscles which lie on the fore-arm—these are for the more powerful actions ; but in the palm of the hand, and between the metacarpal bones, there are small muscles (*Lumbricales and Interossei*), which perform the finer motions, expanding the fingers and moving them in every direction, with great quickness and delicacy. These are the organs which give the hand the power of spinning, weaving, engraving ; and as they produce the quick motions of the musician's fingers, they are called by the anatomist *fidicinales*. Attention to our most common actions will shew us, how the division into fingers, by combining motion with the sense of touch, adapts the hand to grasp, to feel, and to compare. We shall presently see how well the points of the fingers are provided for feeling : as the joints and numerous muscles of the hand are adapted for various, distinct, or separate motions.

In this sketch we have the bones of the paw of the adult Chimpanzee, from Borneo ; and the remarkable peculiarity is the smallness of the thumb; it extends no further than to the root of the fingers. On the length, strength, free lateral motion, and perfect mobility of the thumb, depends the power of the human hand.* The thumb is called *pollex,* because of its strength; and that strength is necessary to the

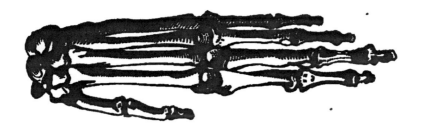

power of the hand, being equal to that of all the fingers. Without the fleshy ball of the thumb, the power of the fingers would avail nothing; and, accordingly, the large ball, formed by the muscles of the thumb, is the distinguishing character of the human hand, and especially of that of an expert workman.†

In a French book, intended to teach young people philosophy, the pupil asks why the fingers are not of equal length? The form of the argument reminds us of the difficulty of putting natural questions—the fault of books of dialogue. However, the master makes the scholar grasp a ball of ivory, to shew him that the points of the fingers are then equal! It would have been better had he closed the fingers upon the palm, and then have asked whether or not they corresponded. This difference in the length of the fingers serves a thousand purposes, adapting the hand and fingers, as in holding a rod, a switch, a sword, a hammer, a pen, or pencil, engraving tool, &c., in all which, a secure hold and freedom of

* The monkey has no separate *flexor longus* of the thumb. Vicq. d'Azyr.

† "*Manus parva, majori adjutrix.*" Albinus.

motion are admirably combined. Nothing is more remarkable, as forming a part of the prospective design to prepare an instrument fitted for the various uses of the human hand, than the manner in which the delicate and moving apparatus of the palm and fingers is guarded. The power with which the hand grasps, as when a sailor lays hold to raise his body in the rigging, would be too great for the texture of mere tendons, nerves, and vessels; they would be crushed, were not every part that bears the pressure, defended with a cushion of fat, as elastic as that which we have described in the foot of the horse and the camel. To add to this purely passive defence, there is a muscle which runs across the palm and more especially supports the cushion on its inner edge. It is this muscle which, raising the edge of the palm, adapts it to lave water, forming the cup of Diogenes.

In conclusion,—what says Ray,—"Some animals "have horns, some have hoofs, some teeth, some ta- "lons, some claws, some spurs and beaks; man hath "none of all these, but is weak and feeble, and sent "unarmed into the world—Why, a hand, with reason "to use it, supplies the use of all these."

CHAPTER IV.

OF THE MUSCLES.

THE muscle of the body is that fleshy part, with which every one is familiar. It consists of fibres which lie parallel to each other. This fibrous, or filamentous part, has a living endowment, a power of contraction and relaxation, termed irritability. A single muscle is formed of some millions of these fibres combined together, having the same point of attachment or origin, and concentrating in a rope or tendon, which is fixed to a moveable part, called its insertion. We may demonstrate upwards of fifty muscles of the arm and hand, all of which must consent to the simplest action; but this gives an imperfect view of the extent of the relation of parts which is necessary to every act of volition. We are most sensible of this combination in the muscles, when inflammation has seized any of the great joints of the body; for even when in bed, every motion of an extremity gives pain, through the necessity of a corresponding movement in the trunk. When we stand, we cannot raise or extend the arm without a new position of the body, and a poising of it, through the action of a hundred muscles.

ON THE ACTION OF THE MUSCLES OF THE ARM.

We shall consider this subject under two heads; in the first, we shall give examples of the living property of the muscles; and then of the mechanical contrivances, in their form and application. In all

8*

that regards the muscles, we see the most bountiful
supply of power commensurate to the object, but
never any thing in the least degree superabundant.
If the limb is to be moved by bringing a muscle, or a
set of muscles into action, the power is not given in
that excess which would enable them to overcome
their opponents ; but the property of action is withdrawn from the opponents; they become relaxed,
and the muscles, which are in a state of contraction,
perform their office with comparative ease. A stationary condition of the limb results from a balanced
but regulated action of all the muscles ; which condition may be called their tone.   If, in an experiment,
a weight be attached to the tendon of an extensor
muscle, it will draw out that muscle to a certain
degree, until its tone or permanent state resists the
weight : but if the flexor muscle be now excited, this
being the natural opponent of the extensor, the
weight will fall, by the relaxation of the extensor.
So that the motion of a limb implies an active state
or a change in both classes of muscles, the one to
contract, the other to relax ; and the will influences
both classes. Were it not so regulated, instead of
the natural, easy, and elegant motions of the frame,
the attempt at action would exhibit the body con-
vulsed, or, as the physicians term it, in clonic spasms.
The similitude of the two sawyers, mentioned by
Paley, gives but an imperfect idea of the adjustment
of the two classes of muscles. When two men are
sawing a log of wood, they pull alternately, and
when the one is pulling, the other resigns all exertion.
But this is not the condition of the muscles—the
relaxing muscle has not given up all effort, like a
loose rope, but it is controlled in its yielding, with as
fine a sense of adjustment, as is the action of the
contracting muscles. Nothing appears to us more
simple than raising the arm, or pointing with the
finger ; yet in that single act, not only are innume-
rable muscles put into activity, but as many are

thrown out of action, and the condition of these
classes is totally opposite to each other, under the
same act of volition.

By such considerations, we are prepared to admire
the faculty which shall combine a hundred muscles
so as to produce a change of posture or action of the
body ; and we now perceive that the power taken
from one class of our muscles, may be considered as
if it were bestowed on the other ; so that the property of life, which we call the irritability, or action
of a muscle, is upon the whole, less exhausted than
would be the case on any other supposition.

As to the second head, our demonstration is of an
easier kind. We have said that nature bestows abundantly, but not superfluously ; a truth evinced in the
arrangement of the muscles. All the muscles of the
limbs have their fibres running in an oblique direction,—thus, A. being the tendinous origin of a muscle,
and B. the tendinous insertion, the fleshy fibres run
obliquely between these two tendons.

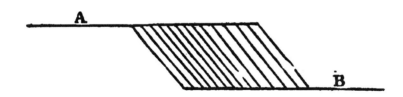

The fibre acting thus obliquely loses power, but
gains the property of pulling what is attached to its
further extremity through a greater space, while it
contracts. This mechanical arrangement is intelli-
gible on the law, that velocity of motion through
space, is equal to power or weight. Here in the
muscle, there is a resignation of power to obtain velocity of motion.

The same effect is produced by the manner in
which the tendons of the muscles run over the joints.
They would act more powerfully, if they went in a

straight line to the toes or tips of the fingers: but
by being laced down in sheaths, they move the toes
and fingers with a velocity proportioned to their loss
of power.   Let us see how far this corresponds with
other mechanical contrivances.   A certain power of
wind or water being obtained, the machinery is
moved; but it is desired to give a blow, with a velocity far greater than the motion of the water or the
turning of the wheels.   For this purpose a fly-wheel
is put on, the spokes of which may be considered as
long levers.   The wheel moves very slowly, at first,
but being once in motion, each impulse accelerates it
with more and more facility; at length, it acquires a
rapidity, and a centrifugal force which nothing can
equal in its effects, but the explosion of gunpowder.
The mechanist not having calculated the power of
the accelerated motion in a heavy wheel, has seen
his machinery split and burst up, and the walls of
the house blown out as by the bursting of a bomb-
shell.   A body at rest receives an impulse from another, which puts it into motion—it receives a second
blow; now, this second blow has much greater effect
than the first—for the power of the first was exhausted in changing the body from a state of rest to
that of motion—but being in motion when it receives
the second blow, the whole power is bestowed on the
acceleration of its motion; and so on, by the third
and fourth blows, until the body moves with a velocity, equal to that of the body from which the impulse is originally given.   The slight blow given to
a boy's hoop is sufficient to keep it running; and just
 so the fly-wheel of a machine is kept in rapid action
by a succession of impulses, each of which would
hardly put it in motion.   If we attempt to stop the
wheel, it will give a blow in which a hundred lesser
impulses are combined and multiplied.

There is, in the machinery of the animal body, in
a lesser degree, the same interchange of velocity
and force.   When a man strikes with a hammer, the

muscle near the shoulder,* c. acts upon the humerus,
B. in raising the extended lever of the arm and
hammer, with every possible disadvantage; seeing
that it is inserted or attached so near the centre of
motion in the shoulder joint.

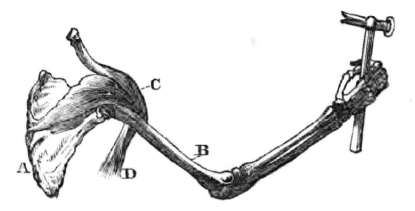

But the loss of power is restored in another form.
What the muscle D. loses by the mode of its insertion,
is made up in the velocity communicated to the hammer; for in descending through a large space, it ac-
cumulates velocity, and velocity is equal to force.—
The advantage of the rapid descent of a heavy body
is, that a smart blow is given, and an effect produced
which the combined power of all the muscles, without this mechanical distribution of force, could not
accomplish. This is, in truth, similar to the operation of the fly wheel, by which the gradual motion of
an engine is accumulated in a point of time, and a
blow is struck capable of crushing or of stamping a
piece of gold or silver. In what respect does the mechanism of the arm differ from the engine with
which the printer throws off his sheet? Here is a
lever with a heavy ball at the end; in proportion to
its weight, it is difficult to be put in motion. The

* A. The scapula, or shoulder blade: B. the humerus, or arm-
bone; c. the deltoid muscle of the shoulder, arising from the shoulder-
blade and clavicle, and inserted into the arm-bone; D. a muscle
which draws the arm down, as in striking with a sword or hammer.

printer, therefore, takes hold of the lever near the ball, at A. Were he to continue pulling at that part of the lever, he would give to the ball no more velocity than that of his hand; but having put the ball into motion, he slips his hand down the lever to B. He could

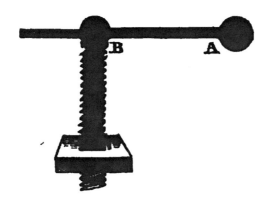

not have moved the weight, had he applied his hand here at first; but it being now in motion, the whole strength of his arm is given to the lever at B., whilst the velocity of the great weight at the further end is accelerated. Thus the weight and the velocity being combined, the impulse given to the screw is much greater than if he had continued to pull upon the further end of the lever at A.

If we now turn our eye to the diagram (page 93), we shall understand that the muscle c. raises the long lever of the arm at a disadvantage, or very slowly; but the arm being moved, that motion is rapidly increased by each successive impulse from the muscle; and, of course, the velocity of the further extremity is more rapid than at the insertion of the tendon.

Again, if we consider the action of the muscle D. in pulling down the arm, as in giving a back stroke with the sword, we have the combination of two powers,—weight and muscular effort. When the hammer descends, the rapidity is increased by the mere effect of gravity; but when the action of the muscle is conjoined, the two forces, progressively increasing, greatly augment the velocity of the descent.

The same interchange of power for velocity, which takes place in the arm, adapts a man's hand and fingers to a thousand arts, requiring quick or lively motions. The fingers of a lady, playing on the pianoforte, or the compositor with his types, are instances of the advantage gained by this sacrifice of force for velocity of movement. The spring of the foot and toe is bestowed in the same manner, and gives elasticity and rapidity in running, dancing, and leaping.

After the many illustrations from mechanics which we have offered, the muscular power itself must be a subject of surprise and admiration. Gravity, the running of water, the expansion and condensation of steam, the production of gases, the spring or elasticity of material, or all these combined, could not have answered the varied offices performed by this one property of life possessed by the muscles. The irritable and contractile fibre, matter which, chemically considered, does not differ from the fibrine of the blood, being endowed with this property of contraction, and adapted with "mechanical ingenuity," fulfils a thousand distinct purposes, in volition, breathing, speaking, in digestion, assimilation, circulation; and in all these it is modified to the wants and condition of every class of animals.

From what the reader already understands of the conformity which subsists among all the parts of an animal body, he will readily comprehend that there is a perfect relation between the bones and the muscles: that as the bones change, and exhibit a variety in their size, relative position, and articulations, so there is an adaptation of the muscles. We sometimes find them separated into smaller muscles, and sometimes consolidated into more powerful masses.

The demonstration to the anatomical student of the muscles of the human hand and arm, becomes the test of his master's perfection as a teacher. Nothing is more uninteresting, tedious, and difficult to attend to, than the demonstration of the muscles of the arm, when they are taken successively, as they present themselves; but when they are taught with lucid arrangement, according to the motions performed by them, it .is positively agreeable to find how much interest may be given to the subject.

It would be foreign to the object of this work to introduce such demonstrations here.

Yet it is very remarkable that the muscles of the arm and hand should resemble so closely the muscles of the fore extremity of the lion, for example. The flexors, extensors, pronators, and supinators are, in the brute, exactly in the same place, and bear all the relations which the student of anatomy is taught to observe with so much interest in the human arm. This example is sufficient to show how accurately the comparative anatomy of the muscles conforms to that of the bones; and that in proportion as the bones of the extremity resemble in shape and power of motion those of the human arm, so do the muscles— another proof of the great extent of the system of relations established in the animal system.

There is one circumstance more which should not be omitted in the comparative anatomy of these muscles, as it exhibits another instance of conformity in their structure, to the offices which they have to perform. We have just stated that the power of contraction is a vital property. The continued action of a muscle, therefore, exhausts the vitality; and to support that action, when it is inordinate, there must be a more than usual provision for the supply of this living power, viz :—a means of increasing or perpetuating the circulation of the blood, which is the source of all vital power.

In the *lemur tardigradus* it has been observed that the axillary and femoral arteries, the great arteries of the anterior and posterior extremities, have this peculiarity—that the trunk is subdivided into a number of equal-sized cylinders, which again unite to form a single trunk previous to the distribution of its branches to the muscles.* It has been argued that this peculiarity, as it produces a retardation of the blood, is adapted to long continued action in the muscles. I believe it to be a provision for long continued action ; because the animals which possess it, are not more remarkable for the slowness of their progression than for the tenacity of their hold. The extremities are long and the muscles powerful, either to sustain the animal by grasping the branches of trees, or for digging ; but surely the strength of the muscles cannot be produced by retardation of the circulation, on the principle, universally admitted, that the expenditure of arterial blood is in proportion to the vital force employed.

Were the arteries of the living body like rigid tubes, and the laws of the circulation the same as those of hydraulics, such might be the conclusion. But it is impossible to suppose that the circulation of the blood could be performed according to the laws which govern the flow of water in dead tubes. The artery is dilatable, it contracts with a vital force ; both the dilatability and the contractility of arteries are subject to the influences of the living principle. When, therefore, the artery of a limb is divided into four or five vessels, the result is a greater capacity of dilatation, a greater power of contraction ; and these being vital operations, are subject to be influenced and adjusted according to the necessity for the increase or diminution of the circulation.

If such a peculiarity in the form of the vessels in the extremities of these animals, retards the blood, it can only be during repose ; for, on excitement, so far from retarding, it must bestow remarkable power of acceleration. I conclude, therefore, that this va-

* There is some doubt as to the reunion of the vessels.

9

riety of distribution in the arteries is a provision for occasional great activity in the muscles of the limb, and for forcing the blood into contact with the fibres, notwithstanding their continued action and rigidity.

We have seen in the preceding chapter the same organ, which moves at one time as slowly as the hand of a watch, at another moves with extreme rapidity : consequently, we cannot admit the inference that the tortuous and subdivided artery is a provision for languid motions.

In speaking of the arteries which go to the hand, it may be expected that we should touch on a subject, which has been formerly a good deal discussed, whether the properties of the right hand, in comparison with those of the left, depend on the course of the arteries to it. It is affirmed that the trunk of the artery going to the right arm, passes off from the heart so as to admit the blood directly and more forcibly into the small vessels of the arm. This is assigning a cause which is unequal to the effect, and presenting, altogether, too confined a view of the subject : it is a participation in the common error of seeking in the mechanism the cause of phenomena which have a deeper source.

For the conveniences of life, and to make us prompt and dexterous, it is pretty evident that there ought to be no hesitation which hand is to be used, or which foot is to be put forward ; nor is there, in fact, any such indecision. Is this taught, or have we this readiness given to us by nature ? It must be observed, at the same time, that there is a distinction in the whole right side of the body, and that the left side is not only the weaker, in regard to muscular strength, but also in its vital or constitutional properties. The developement of the organs of action and motion is greatest upon the right side, as may at any time be ascertained by measurement, or the testimony of the tailor or shoemaker ; certainly, this superiority may be said to result from the more frequent exertion of the right hand; but the peculiarity extends to the constitution also; and disease attacks the left extremities more frequently than the right. In opera dancers, we may see that the most difficult feats are performed by the right foot. But their preparatory exercises better evince the natural weakness of the left limb, since these performers are made to give double practice to it, in order to avoid awkwardness in the public exhibition; for if these exercises be neglected, an ungraceful preference will be given to the right side. In walking behind a person, it is very seldom that we see an equalized motion of the body; and if we look to the left foot, we shall find that the tread is not so firm upon it, that the toe is not so much turned out as in the right, and that a greater push is made with it. From the peculiar form of woman, and the elasticity of her step resulting more from the motion of the ankle than of the haunches, the defect of the left foot when it exists, is more apparent in her gait. No boy hops upon his left foot, unless he be left handed. The horseman puts the left foot in the stirrup and springs from the right. We think we may conclude, that every thing being adapted in the conveniences of life to the right hand, as for example the direction of the worm of the screw or of the cutting end of the auger, is not arbitrary, but is related to a natural endowment of the body. He who is left handed is most sensible to the advantages of this adaptation, from the opening of the parlour-door to the opening of a pen-knife. On the whole, the preference of the right hand is not the effect of habit, but is a natural provision, and is bestowed for a very obvious purpose: and the property does not depend on the peculiar distribution of the arteries of the arm—but the preference is given to the right foot, as well as to the right hand.

CHAPTER V.

THE SUBSTITUTION OF OTHER ORGANS FOR THE HAND.

AFTER having examined the manner in which one instrument, the hand, is modified and adapted to a variety of purposes in different animals, there remains only this mode of elucidation—that we contrast it with its imperfect substitutes in other creatures. I might, indeed, have shewn in the insect tribes the most curious examples of instruments for similar purposes with the hand and fingers of man; but I have intentionally confined this inquiry to the higher classes of animals.

The habits of some fishes require that they should cling firmly to the rocks or to whatever presents to them. There locomotive powers are perfect; but how are they to become stationary in the tide or the stream? I have often thought it wonderful that the salmon or the trout, for example, should keep its place, night and day, in the rapid current. In the sea, there are some fishes especially provided with means of clinging to the rocks. The lumpfish, *cyclopterus lumpus*, fastens itself by an apparatus which is on the lower part of its body. The sucking fish, *remora*, has a similar provision on its back. It attaches itself to the surface of the shark and to whatever is afloat; and, of course, to the bottoms of ships. The ancients believed it capable of stopping a ship under sail, and Pliny, therefore, called it remora. We must admire the means by which these fishes retain their proper position in the water, without clinging by their fins or teeth, and while they are free for such efforts as enable them* to seize their food. The apparatus by which they attach themselves resembles a boy's sucker : the organ being pressed against the surface to which the creature is to be fixed, the centre is drawn by muscles in the same manner that the sucker is drawn with the cord, and thus a vacuum is made.

In the cuttle-fish we see a modification of this apparatus : the suckers are on the extremities of their processes or arms, and become instruments of prehension and of locomotion. They are capable of turning in all directions, either to fix the animal or to drag it from place to place. In the Indian Seas, these creatures become truly terrific from the length of their arms, which extend to eight or nine fathoms, and from the firmness with which they cling.

Dr. Shaw tells us, that on throwing a fish of the species cyclopterus lumpus into a pail of water, it fixed itself so firmly to the bottom, that by taking hold of the tail, he lifted up the pail, although it contained some gallons of water.

There is another fish, which from its name we should expect to perform strange antics ; it is called harlequin angler.[†] It appearance is grotesque and singular ; the pectoral fins resemble short arms, and are palmated at their tips.[‡] M. Renau, in his histo-

---

* In the Mollusca and Zoophytes we find many instances of the animal holding on against the force of tide or current. The Actiniæ fix themselves to rocks and shells ; and some, as the sea carnation, hang suspended from the lower surface of projecting rocks, resembling the calyx of a flower. By the elongation of their tentacula, they expand and blow out like a flower; but instead of petals, these are prehensile instruments by which they draw whatever food floats near them into their stomachs. The Byssus of the muscle is a set of filaments which retains the shell at anchor and prevents it drifting or rolling with the tide. These filaments are the secretion of a gland, and whilst they are fixed to the rock, the gland retains the hold at their other ends. The shell of the oyster is itself cemented to the rock.

† *Lophius Histrio*, from a Greek word that has reference to the process which floats from the head, like a streamer or pennant.

‡ These fins have two bones in them like the radius and ulna ; but Cuvier says, that they are more strictly bones of the carpus.

ry of fishes, affirms that he knew an individual of this species; and the expression is not so incorrect, since he saw it for three days out of the water, walking about the house in the manner of a dog. The circumstance of its walking out of the water has some interest, as showing relations between organs which are apparently the least connected. The fact of this fish living out of the water is doubted; but the form of its branchial organs inclines me to believe it; and its habits require such a provision. In this genus, the operculum does not open to let the respired water pass off freely behind, as in most fishes; but the water is discharged by a small aperture which, in Mr. Owen's opinion, is capable of being closed by a sphincter. The cavities in which the branchiæ lie are large, and this is, indeed, partly the reason of the monstrous head of this fish. Thus, it has not only its fins converted into feet, but its gills into pouches, capable of containing water, and of permitting the function of the branchiæ to proceed when the water is retired; that is, when it lies in mud, or shallow pools; for in such situations does the lophius find its food, where it angles for it in a very curious manner.

But there are other fishes that move out of the water on dry land, and even ascend trees, without being carried there by floods. The *perca scandens*, by means of the spines of its gill-covers, and the spinous rays of its fins, climbs trees; so that Dr. Shaw calls it the climbing fish.*

All creatures which have their skins protected, whether by feathers, or shells, or scales, have an exquisite touch in their mouth, or in the appendages which hang from it. Fishes have *cirri* which hang from their mouth, and these are equivalent to the palpa and tentacula of insects and crustacea. The

---

* The spines of the Echinus are moveable; they assist in progression. They are directed towards an advancing enemy! Although these spines may be effectual for their purpose they are the lowest or least perfect substitutes for the extremities.

fishing lines of the *lophius piscatorius* are examples of these processes : and Pliny relates that this frog-like fish, hiding in the mud, leaves the extremities of these filaments visible; which, from their resemblance to worms, entice the smaller fishes, and they become the prey of their concealed enemy. It is surprising how varied the means are by which fishes obtain their food. The *chætodon* (bandouliere à bec) squirts water at flies as they pass and brings them down. The *sciæna jaculatrix*, according to Pallas, has a similar power; and the *sparus insidiator* catches aquatic insects by the sudden projection of its snout. It is affirmed by some naturalists that the rays of the dorsal and anal fins, as in the cordonnier of Martinique, *zeus ciliaris*, le blepharis, Cuv., are employed to grapple or coil round the stems of plants and sustain the fish.

The several offices attributed to these processes in fishes imply that they possess sensibility, if not muscular power.

By anatomical investigation and experiment, I, some years ago, discovered that the sensibility of all the head and of its various appendages resulted from one nerve only of the ten which are enumerated as arising from the brain, and are distributed within and around the head; and, pursuing the subject by the aid of comparative anatomy, I found that a nerve corresponding to this, which is the fifth nerve in man, served a similar purpose in all the lower animals. In creatures which are covered with feathers or scales, or protected by shell, this nerve becomes almost the sole organ of sensibility. It is the developement of this nerve which gives sensibility to the cirri, which hang about the mouths of fishes, and to the palpa of the crustacea and insects. It is the same nerve which supplies the tongue, and is the organ of its exquisite sensibility to touch, as well as of taste. In some animals, especially in the reptiles, the tongue, by its length and mobility, becomes a substitute for these external appendages.   We might have noticed before, that the tongue is an organ of prehension as well as of touch.   With it the ox gathers in the herbage ; and in the giraffe, it is rather curious to observe that as the whole frame of the animal is calculated to raise the head to a great height, so is the tongue capable of projecting beyond the mouth to an extraordinary extent, to wrap round and pull down the extreme branches of trees.   The whiskers of the feline quadrupeds possess a fine sensibility through branches of the fifth nerve, which enter their roots.   Birds have a high degree of sensibility to touch in their mouths.   In ducks, and all that quaffer with their bills under water, the sense is very fine, and we find, on dissection, that a branch of the fifth nerve, remarkably developed, is distributed on the upper mandible. Animals feel in the whole of their external surface ; and we may say that serpents, by coiling themselves round a body, have the organ of touch all over them. Still the fifth pair of nerves in the head, or the nerve analogous to it, is the main instrument of touch in the greater number of animals where extremities are wanting.   There are organs varying in their conformation, sometimes delicate palpa, sometimes horny rods, and these are often possessed of muscularity as well as sensibility; but to all, the sense of touch is bestowed through a nerve corresponding with the fifth pair, the nerve of the tongue and lips, and of the muscles of the jaws in man.

But we may repeat, that, necessary as these appendages and this sensibility are to the existence of these animals, their imperfections serve, by contrast, 'to show how happily the different properties are combined in the hand ; in which we perceive the sensibilities to changes of temperature, to touch, and to motion, united with a facility in the joints of unfolding and moving in every possible degree and direction, without abruptness or angularity, and in a manner inimitable by any artifice of joints and levers.

CHAPTER VI.

THE ARGUMENT PURSUED FROM THE COMPARATIVE ANATOMY.

So far as we have hitherto proceeded, by examining objects in comparative anatomy which from their magnitude can not be misunderstood, we have been led to conclude that, independently of the system of parts marvellously combined to form the individual animal, there is another, more comprehensive system, which embraces all animals; and which exhibits a certain uniformity in the functions of life, however different in form or bulk the creatures may be, or to whatever condition of the globe they may have been adapted. We have seen no accidental deviation or deformity, but that every change has been for a purpurpose, and every part has had its just relation. We have witnessed all the varieties moulded to such a perfect accommodation, and the alterations produced by such minute degrees, that all notion of external and accidental agency must be rejected.

We might carry our demonstration downward through the lower classes of animals; for example, we might trace the feet of insects from their most perfect or complex state, till they disappear; or, observing the changes in another direction, we might follow out the same parts from the smallest beginning to the most perfect condition of the member, where we see the thigh, leg, and tarsus of the fly. We might distinguish them at first as the fine cirri, like minute bristles, which on the bodies of worms take slight hold of the surface over which they creep. In the sea mouse, (*aphrodita*) we might notice these

bristles standing out from distinct mammillary processes, which are furnished with appropriate muscles.
Then in the *myriapodes*, the first order of insects, we
might see the same " many feet," and each foot
having a distinct articulation.   From that, we might
pass to the feet of those insects, where there is a thigh,
leg, and foot, with the most perfect system of flexors,
extensors, and adductor muscles, possessing, in fine,
all that we most admire in the human anatomy.
Nay, it is most curious to observe how the feet of the
true insects are again changed or modified ; taking
new offices, the anterior feet becoming feelers, organs
of prehension, or *hands*.   When, with such an object, we view the delicate and curiously adapted instruments of insects, we must perceive that it would
be easy to trace almost every part through a succession of modifications.   Among the *vertebrata*, we have
seen the hand become a wing or a fin ; so might we
trace the wings of insects.   If we begin with a fly,
which has two delicate and perfect wings incased
and protected, we find that the covers are raised to
admit the expansion of the wings.   In another, the
case becomes a wing ; and the fly is characterized
by four wings.   Proceed to examine a third example,
and we shall discover that this anterior wing is larger
and more perfect than the posterior : the fourth specimen has lost the posterior wings, and has only two
perfect ones ; and if we continue the examination,
the next specimen will present an insect deprived of
wings altogether.   These are not freaks of nature,
but new forms of the body ; new appendages required for a different poising of the fly in its flight.
They are adaptations in that regular series which
we have observed to obtain in the larger animals,
and where the intention can not be mistaken.
A very natural question will force itself upon us, how
are those varieties to be explained ?

The curious adaptation of a member to different
offices and to different conditions of the animal has

led to a very extraordinary opinion in the present day,—that all animals consist of the same elements. It would be just to say that they consist of the same chemical elements, and that they attract and assimilate matter by the performance of the same vital functions, through every species of animals, however different in form and structure. But by the elements which are now mentioned, the authors of this new theory mean certain pieces which enter into the structure of the body, and which they illustrate by the analogy of the building materials of a house. If these materials, they say, are exhausted in the ornamental parts of the portico and vestibule, there must be a proportionate limitation of the apartments for the family !

This new theory has been brought forward with the highest pretensions; the authors of it have called upon us to mark the moment of its conception as the commencement of a new æra ! They speak of the "elective affinities of organs," "the balancing of organs," "a new principle of connection," and a "new theory of analysis."—The hypothesis essentially is this, that when a part, which belongs to one animal, is missed in another, we are to seek for it in some neighbouring organ: and on such grounds they affirm, that this surpasses all former systems as a means of discovery. Now, the perfection or aggrandizement of any one organ of an animal is not attended with the curtailment or proportional deficiency of any other. Like ourselves, perhaps, the supporters of this theory dwell too much upon the bones; but even in them, we shall show that the system is untenable. In the mean time, we may ask, do additional parts connected with the stomach, making it highly complex, as in ruminating animals, shorten the intestinal canal, or make its form simpler ? On the contrary, is not a complex stomach necessarily connected with a long and complicated intestine ?— Does a complex intestinal canal throughout all its

course render imperfect the solid viscera which are
in juxtaposition to it? Is there any defect in them,
because the organs of digestion are perfect, or complicated? Does the complex heart imply a more
simple, or a more perfect condition of the lungs? In
short, as animals rise in the scale of existence, do we
not find that the systems of digestion, circulation, respiration and sensation, bear ever a proportional increase? Is there any instance of an improvement in
one organ thrusting another out of its place, or diminishing its volume?

Now, as to the osseous system, were we to follow
these theorists into the very stronghold of their position, the bones of the skull, where the real intricacy
of the parts allows them some scope for their ingenuity, we might show how untenable the principle is
which they assume. But we must confine ourselves
to our own subject.

In the higher orders of the vertebrata, we find that
the bones of the shoulder perform a double office;
that they have an important share in the act of respiration, whilst they are perfect as a foundation for
the extremity. Now, let us take an instance where
the mode of respiration of the animal is inconsistent
with what we may term the original mechanism of
the bones of the shoulder. In the batrachian order,
the ribs are wanting: where then are we to look for
them? Shall we follow a system which informs us
that when a bone is wanting in the cavity of the ear,
we are to seek for it in the jaw; and which, yet, shall
leave us in the contemplation of this class of animals deficient in thirty-two ribs, without pointing out
where they are to be found, or how their elements are
built up in other structures? If, on the contrary,
we take the principle that parts are formed or withdrawn, with a never-failing relation to the function
which is to be performed, we see that no sooner are
the compages of the chest removed, and the shoulder thus deprived of support, than the bones to which

the extremity is fixed are expanded and varied, both in form and articulation, so as to fulfil their main object of giving security and motion to the arm.

With respect to the instance which we have accidentally noticed regarding the mechanism of the jaw in birds, and which is brought forward so vauntingly as a proof of the excellence of the theory, it does, indeed, prove the reverse of what is assumed. The only effect of this hypothesis is to make us lose sight of the principle which ought to direct us in the observation of such curious structures, as well as of the conclusions to which an unbiassed mind would come. The matter to be explained is simply this :—the chain of bones in the ear, which is so curiously adapted in the mammalia to convey the vibrations of the membrane of the tympanum to the nerve of hearing, is not found in the organ of hearing in birds ; but there is substituted a mechanism entirely different. They choose to say that the incus, one of the bones of the chain, is wanting in the bird. Where shall we find it ?—they ask. Here it is in the apparatus of the jaw or mandible ; in that bone which is called *os quadratum.* I believe that the slight and accidental resemblance which this bone (B.) in the bird has to the incus, is the real origin of this fancy. Let us follow a juster mode of reasoning, and see how this hypothesis obscures the beauty of the subject. The first step of the investigation ought to be to inquire into the fact, if there be any imperfection in the hearing of birds. That is easily answered—the hearing of birds is most acute ; the slightest noise alarms ; and the nightingale, or other bird of song, in a summer evening, will answer to the note of his rival when he is out of our hearing. We have next to observe the imperfection in the organ—the want of an external ear ; which, were it present, would be at variance with all that we have most to admire in the shape of the bird and the direction of the feathers, as conducing to its rapid passage through the air. With this obvious defect of the external ear, can we admit that the internal ear is also imperfect, notwithstanding the very remarkable acuteness of hearing, which we know to result from this internal structure, and from it alone? Now we do, in fact, find a different structure in the ear of birds; but, yet nothing is wanting. The *columella* is a shaft of bone of exquisite delicacy, which is extended from the outward membrane of the ear to the labyrinth or proper seat of the nerve of hearing. It occupies the place and office of the chain of four bones which belong to the ear of mammalia. We have no authority, however, for affirming that the incus is here wanting more than any other bone of the chain;—and if it be said that the os quadratum is the missing incus, why should not we find in the oviparous reptiles, where there is a *columella* in the ear, an os quadratum in the jaw?

From this mode of inquiry, we find that the sense of hearing is enjoyed in an exquisite degree in birds: that the organ of the sense is not imperfect, but is adapted to a new construction, and a varied apparatus—suited to the condition of the bird: and that there is no accidental dislocation or substitution of something less perfect than what we find in other classes of animals.

If we now look to the structure of the mandible of the bird, we shall find as curious, though a somewhat grosser example of mechanical relation. The bill of the bird, in some degree, pertains to our subject, as it is the organ of prehension and of touch. It is withal a fly trap—hence, its motions must be rapid: and the velocity is increased by the most obvious means imaginable,—that is, by giving motion to both mandibles, instead of to one. When a dog snaps he throws back his head, and thereby raises the upper jaw at the same time that the lower jaw is dropped; but these are slow and clumsy motions, pertaining to the muscles of the neck as well as of the jaws, and the poor hound makes many attempts, before he catches the fly that teazes him. But a swallow or fly-catcher makes no second effort, so admirably suited is the apparatus of prehension to the liveliness of the eye and the instinct. The adaptation of the instrument consists in this, that the muscles which open the lower mandible, by the same effort,

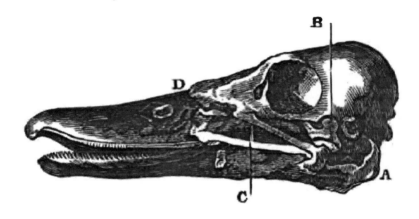

open the upper one : A. is a process of the lower mandible, projecting much behind the centre of motion, and the muscle which is attached to it opens the bill ;—but at the same time, the lower mandible presses upon the bone B., the *os quadratum :* now, there is attached to this bone, projecting forwards, with its anterior extremity fixed against the upper mandible, a shaft or process of bone c. ; and this receives the pressure of the *os quadratum*, when the muscle acts ; so that being thrust forwards, like a bolt, it opens the upper mandible, which moves upon the skull at D. Here, then, is a piece of mechanism as distinct as the lock of a gun, which is for the purpose, as we have said, of giving rapidity to the motions of the bill. Is it nearer the truth to consider this as a new apparatus, suiting the necessities of the creature, or an accidental result of the introduction of a bone, which in its proper office has nothing to do with the jaw?

But we have wandered somewhat from our subject. We have taken the bones of the shoulder, or those of the extremity which are nearest to the trunk; we may pursue the inquiry by noticing those which are most remote from it. In the bones of the hand, we have seen that the same system was variously modified so as to be adapted to every possible change in office. But as it is insisted that the number of parts continue the same, what can we say to the bones of the paddle in the saurian and chelonian tribes, which, as in the ichthyosaurus for example, consist of sixty or seventy polygonous bones; whilst in the horse there are only fifteen bones; and in man, twenty-seven. Yet, with all those bones in the paddle, there is still the full complement in the part that corresponds with the arm. If the system fail us in such an obvious instance as this, with what confidence can we prosecute the intricate bones of the spine and head under its guidance?

Seeking assistance from the works of distinguished naturalists, we do not always find that disposition of mind prevail, which we should be apt to suppose a necessary result of their peculiar studies. We do not discover that combination of genius with sound sense, which distinguished Cuvier, and the great men of science. It is, above all, surprising with what perverse ingenuity men seek to obscure the conception of a Divine Author, an intelligent, designing, and benevolent Being—rather clinging to the greatest absurdities, or interposing the cold and inanimate influence of the mere elements, in a manner to extinguish all feeling of dependance in our minds, and all emotions of gratitude.

Some will maintain that all the varieties which we see, are the result of a change of circumstances influencing the original animal; or that new organs have been produced by a desire and consequent effort of the animal to stretch and mould itself—that, as the leaves of a plant expand to light, or turn to the sun, or as the roots shoot to the appropriate soil, so do the exterior organs of animals grow and adapt themselves. We shall presently find that an opinion has prevailed that the organization of animals determines their propensities; but the philosophers, of whom we are now speaking, imagine the contrary,—that under the influence of new circumstances, organs have accommodated themselves, and assumed their particular forms.

It must be here remarked that there are no instances of the production of new organs by the union of individuals belonging to different species. Nor is there any foundation in observation for the opinion that a new species may be formed by the union of individuals of different families. But it is contended, that, although the species of animals have not changed in the last 5000 years, we do not know what might have been the effect of the revolution before that time; that is, previous to the present condition of the world. But, on subjects of this nature, we must argue from what we know, and from what we see.

We do perceive surprising changes in the conformation of animals; some of them are very familiar to us; but all show a foreknowledge and a prospective plan, an alteration gradually taking place in preparation for the condition, never consequent upon it. It will be sufficient for our purpose, if we take the highest and the lowest examples. Man has two conditions of existence in the body. Hardly two creatures can be less alike than an infant and a man. The whole fœtal state is a preparation for birth. My readers would not thank me, were I to show how necessary all the proportions and forms of the infant are to his being born alive,—and yet nothing is so easy to demonstrate. Every one may see that from the moment of birth there is a new impulse given to the growth, so as finally to adapt the proportions of the body to the state of perfect manhood. Few, however, are aware that the fœtus has a *life* adapted

10*

to its condition, and that if the confinement of the womb were protracted beyond the appointed time, it must die !—from no defect of nourishment, but simply, because the time is come for a change in its whole economy !

Now, during all the long period of gestation, the organs are forming; the lungs are perfected before the admission of air—new tubes are constructed before the flood-gates, which are to admit the blood, are opened. But there are finer, and more curious, provisions than these. If we take any of the grand organs, as the heart, or the brain, and examine it through all its gradations of change in the embryo state, we shall recognize it simple, at first, and gradually developing, and assuming the peculiarities which finally distinguish it. So that it is affirmed, and not without the support of a most curious series of observations, that the human brain, in its earlier stage, resembles that of a fish : as it is developed, it resembles more the cerebral mass of the reptile ; in its increase, it is like that of a bird, and slowly, and only after birth, does it assume the proper form and consistence of the human encephalon. But in all these changes to which man is subject, we nowhere see the influence of the elements, or any other cause than that it has been so predestined. And if, passing over the thousand instances which might be gathered from the intermediate parts of the chain of animal existence, we take the lowest link, and look to the metamorphosis of insects, the conclusion will be the same.

For example, if we examine the larva of a winged insect, we shall see the provisions for its motion over the ground, in that condition, all admirably supplied in the arrangement of its muscles, and the distribution of its nervous system. But if, anticipating its metamorphosis, we dissect the same larva immediately before the change, we shall find a new apparatus in progress towards perfection ; the muscles of its many feet are seen decaying ; the nerves to each muscle are wasting; a new arrangement of muscles, with new points of attachment, directed to the wings instead of the feet, is now visible; and a new distribution of nerves is distinctly to be traced, accommodated to the parts which are now to be put in motion. Here is no budding and stretching forth under the influence of the surrounding elements; but a change operated on all the economy, and prospective, that is, in reference to a condition which the creature has not yet attained.

These facts countenance the conclusion drawn from the comparative anatomy of the hand and arm—that with each new instrument, visible externally, there are a thousand internal relations established: a mechanical contrivance in the bones and joints, which alters every part of the skeleton: an arrangement of muscles, in just correspondence: a texture of nervous filaments, which is laid intermediate between the instrument and the very centre of life and motion; and, finally, as we shall discover from what follows, new sources of activity must be created in relation to the new organ, otherwise the part will hang a useless appendage.

It must now be apparent that nothing less than the Power, which originally created, is equal to the effecting of those changes on animals, which are to adapt them to their conditions: that their organization is predetermined, and not consequent on the condition of the earth or the surrounding elements. Neither can a property in the animal itself account for the changes which take place in the individual, any more than for the varieties which take place in the species. Every thing declares the species to have its origin in a distinct creation, not in a gradual variation from some original type; and any other hypothesis than that of a new creation of animals suited to the successive changes in the inorganic matter of the globe—the condition of the water, atmosphere, and temperature—brings with it only an accumulation of difficulties.

CHAPTER VII.

OF SENSIBILITY AND TOUCH.

WE find every organ of sense, with the exception of that of touch, more perfect in brutes than in man. In the eagle and the hawk, in the gazelle and in the feline tribe, the perfection of the eye is admirable;— in the dog, wolf, hyæna, as well as in birds of prey, the sense of smelling is inconceivably acute; and if we should have some hesitation in assigning a more exquisite sense of taste to brutes, we cannot doubt the superiority of that of hearing in the inferior animals. But in the sense of touch, seated in the hand, man claims the superiority; and it is of consequence to our conclusion that we should observe why it is so.

It has been said that, accompanying the exercise of touch, there is a desire of obtaining knowledge; in other words, a determination of the will towards the organ of the sense. Bichat says, it is active whilst the other senses are passive. This opinion implies that there is something to be understood—something deeper than what is here expressed. We shall arrive at the truth by considering that in the use of the hand there is a double sense exercised; we must not only feel the contact of the object, but we must be sensible to the muscular effort which is made to reach it, or to grasp it in the fingers. It is in the exercise of this latter power that there is really an effort made; there is no more direction of the will towards the nerve of touch, than towards any other sensible nerve. But, before entering on the consideration of the sensibility and action which belong to the fingers, we must attend to the common sensibility of the surface.

Besides that the common sensibility belongs to the hand, and that some inquiry into it is necessary to the completion of our subject, I pursue it the more willingly, because there is no other which affords more surprising proofs of design and of benevolence in the Author of our being. However obvious the proofs may be which are drawn from the mechanism of the body, they are not to be compared with, in this respect, to those which are derived from the living endowments of the frame.

I have used the term common sensibility in conformity with the language of authors and with customary parlance; but the expressions, the "common nerves," and the "common sensibility," in a philosophical inquiry, are inadmissible. Indeed, these terms have been the cause of much of the obscurity which has hung over the subject of the nervous system, and of our blindness to the benevolent adaptation of the endowments of that system to the condition of animal existence. Thus, it has been supposed that some nerves are more coarsely provided for sensation, and that others are of a finer quality, adapted to more delicate impressions. It is assumed that the nerve of the eye is finer than the nerve of the finger—without considering that the retina is insensible to that quality of matter of which we readily acquire the knowledge through touch. Nerves are, indeed, appropriated to peculiar senses, and to the bestowing of distinct functions, but delicacy of texture has nothing to do with this. The nerve of touch in the skin is insensible to light or to sound, not because it has a coarser or more common texture: The beauty and perfection of the system is, that the nerve is made susceptible to its peculiar impression only. The nerve of the skin is alone capable of giving the sense of contact, as the nerve of vision is confined to its own office. If this appropriation resulted merely from a more delicate texture: if the retina were sensible to the matter of light only from possessing a finer sensibility than the nerve of touch, it would be a source of torment; whereas it is most beneficently provided that it shall not be sensible to pain, nor be capable of conveying any impressions to the mind, but those which operate according to its proper function, producing light and colour.

, The pain which we experience in the eye, and the irritation from dust, are owing to a distinct nerve from that of vision, and are consequent on the susceptibility of the surface to a different kind of impression; of which more presently. We should keep in mind the interesting fact, that when surgeons perform the operation of.couching, the point of the needle, in passing through the outer coat of the eye, gives a sensation of pricking, which is an exercise of the nerve of touch; but when the point passes through the retina, which is the expanded nerve of vision and form the internal coat of the eye, the sensation that is produced is as of a spark of fire. The nerve of vision is as insensible to touch as the nerve of touch is to light.*

The extreme sensibility of the skin to the slightest injury conveys to every one the notion—that the pain must be the more severe the deeper the wound. This is not the fact, nor would it accord with the beneficent design which shines out every where. The sensibility of the skin serves not only to give the sense of touch, but it is a guard upon the deeper parts; and as they cannot be reached except through the skin, and we must suffer pain, therefore, before they are injured, it would be superfluous to bestow sensibility upon these deeper parts. If the internal parts which act in the motions of the body had possessed a similar degree

---

* The views of the nervous system, which are shortly given in the text, guided me in my original experiments made twenty-two years ago. They have been attributed to foreign physiologists. The ignorance of what has been done in England, may be, for strangers, an excuse for maintaining these opinions as their own; but the authors at home, who should have known what has been taught in this country, are inexcusable when they countenance these assumptions.

and kind of sensibility with the skin, so far from serving any useful purpose, this sensibility would have
been a source of inconvenience and continual pain in
the common exercise of the frame.

The reason why surgeons more than physicians
have advanced the study of physiology, may be, that
they become practically acquainted with the phenomena on which the science is founded. The surgeon
who has to perform an operation by incision, when he
has cut through the skin, informs his patient that the
greatest pain is over. If, in the advanced stage of
the operation, he has to extend the incision of the skin,
it is very properly considered as a great awkwardness;
and this not only because it proves that he has mis-
calculated what was necessary to the correct performance of his operation, but because the patient, bearing courageously the deeper incisions, cannot sustain
the renewed cutting of the skin, without giving toker
of severe pain.

The fact of the exquisite sensibility of the surface,
in comparison with the deeper parts, being thus ascertained by daily experience, we cannot mistake the
intention : that the skin is made a safeguard to the
delicate textures which are contained within, by
forcing us to avoid injuries: and it does afford us a
more effectual defence than if our bodies were covered
with the hide of the rhinoceros.

The fuller the consideration which we give to this
subject, the more convincing are the proofs that the
painful sensibility of the skin is a benevolent provision, making us alive to those injuries, which, but for
this quality of the nervous system, would bruise and
destroy the internal and vital parts. In pursuing the
inquiry, we learn with much interest that when the
bones, joints, and all the membranes and ligaments
which cover them, are exposed—they may be cut,
pricked, or even burned, without the patient or the
animal, suffering the slightest pain. These facts
must appear to be conclusive ; for who, witnessing

these instances of insensibility, would not conclude
that the parts were devoid of sensation.   But when
we take the true, philosophical, and I may say the
religious view of the subject, and consider that pain
is not an evil, but given for benevolent purposes and
for some important object, we should be unwilling to
terminate the investigation here.

In the first place, we must perceive that if a sensibility similar to that of the skin had been given to
these internal parts, it must have remained unexercised.   Had they been made sensible to pricking and
burning, they would have possessed a quality which
would never have been useful, since no such injuries
can reach them ; or never without warning being
received through the sensibility of the skin.

But, further, if we find that sensibility to pain is a
benevolent provision, and is bestowed for the purpose
of warning us to avoid such violence as would affect
the functions or uses of the parts, we may yet inquire whether any injury can reach these internal
parts without the sensibility of the skin being excited.
Now, of this there can be no doubt, for they are subject to sprain, and rupture, and shocks, without the
skin being implicated in the accident.   If we have
been correct in our inference, there should be a provision to guide us in the safe exercise of the limbs ;
and notwithstanding what has been apparently demonstrated of the insensibility of these internal parts,
they must possess an appropriate sensibility, or it
would imply an imperfection.

With these reflections, we recur to experiment—
and we find that the parts, which are insensible to
pricking, cutting, and burning, are actually sensible
to concussion, to stretching, or laceration.

How consistent, then, and beautiful is the distribution of this quality of life !   The sensibility to pain
varies with the function of the part.   The skin is
endowed with sensibility to every possible injurious
impression which may be made upon it.   But had

this kind and degree of sensibility been made universal, we should have been racked with pain in the common motions of the body : the mere weight of one part on another, or the motion of the joint, would have been attended with that degree of suffering which we experience in using or walking with an inflamed limb.

But on the other hand, had the deeper parts possessed no sensibility, we should have had no guide in our exertions. They have a sensibility limited to the kind of injury which it is possible may reach them, and which teaches us what we can do with impunity. If we leap from too great a height, or carry too great a burthen, or attempt to interrupt a body whose impetus is too great for us, we are warned of the danger as effectually by this internal sensibility, as we are of the approach of a sharp point or a hot iron to the skin.

Returning to the consideration of the sensibility of the skin, in order more fully to comprehend the benevolent effect of it, or in other words, its necessity to our very existence, I may be excused for stating the argument to the reader as I have delivered it in my lectures to the College of Surgeons.

"Without meaning to impute to you inattention or " restlessness, I may request you to observe how every " one occasionally changes his position and shifts the " pressure of the weight of his body ; were you con- " strained to retain one position during the whole " hour, you would rise stiff and lame. The sensi- " bility of the skin is here guiding you to that, which " if neglected, would be followed even by the death " of the part. When a patient has been received " into the hospital with paralysis of the lower part of " the body, we must give especial directions to the " nurse and attendants that the position of his limbs " should be changed at short intervals, that pillows " should be placed under his loins and hams, and that " they should be often shifted. If this be neglected, " you know the consequence to be inflammation of

"the parts that press upon the bed; from which come
"local irritation, then fever and mortification and
"death.

"Thus you perceive that the natural sensibility of
"the skin, without disturbing your train of thought,
"induces you to shift the body so as to permit the free
"circulation of the blood in the minute vessels; and
"that when this sensibility is wanting, the utmost
"attention of friends and the watchfulness of the
"nurse are but a poor substitute for this protection
"which nature is continually affording. If you suf-
"fer thus lying on a soft bed, when deprived of the
"sensibility of the skin, how could you encounter
"without it the rubs and impulses incident to an ac-
"tive life? You must now acknowledge that the
"sensibility of the skin is as much a protection to the
"frame generally, as the sensibility of the eyelids is
"to the eyes, and gives you a motive for gratitude
"which probably you never thought of."

The sensibility of the hand to heat, is a different
endowment from that of touch. This sensibility to
the varieties of temperature is seated in the skin, and
is, consequently, limited to the exterior surface of the
body. The internal parts of the body being of a uniform temperature, it would have been, in them, a
quality altogether superfluous. But as we are surrounded by a temperature continually varying, and
are subject to destruction by its extremes, and as we
must suit our exertions or our contrivances so as to
sustain life against these vicissitudes, our possession
of this peculiar sensibility on the surface affords
another proof of there having been a foreknowledge of our condition. We might, indeed, take
our former example in evidence of what must befal
through the want of this sensibility—the paralytic is
brought to us severely burned, or with his extremities
mortified through cold. A man having lost the sense
of heat in his right hand, but retaining the muscular
power, lifted the cover of a pan which had fallen into

the fire and deliberately replaced it, not being conscious that it was burning hot; the effect, however, was the death and destruction of the skin of the palm and fingers. In this man there was a continual sensation of coldness in the affected arm, which actual cold applied to the extremity did not aggravate nor heat in any degree assuage.* Sensibility to heat is a safeguard in as much as it is capable of becoming a painful sensation, whilst it is a never-failing excitement to activity and a continual source of enjoyment.

And here we may remark an adaptation of the living property very different from the physical influence. Heat is uniform in its effect on matter; but the sensation varies as it is given or abstracted from the living body. Cold and heat are distinct sensations; and this is so far important that without such contrast we should not continue to enjoy the sense. For in the nervous system it holds universally that variety or contrast is necessary to sensation, the finest organ of sense losing its property by the continuance of the same impression. It is by a comparison of cold and heat that we enjoy either condition.

To contrast still more strongly the sensibility of the surface with the property of internal parts, to shew how very different sensibility is, in reality, from what is suggested by first experience, and how admirably it is varied and accommodated to the functions, we shall add one other fact. The brain is insensible —that part of the brain, which if disturbed or diseased, takes away consciousness, is as insensible as the leather of our shoe! That the brain may be touched, or a portion of it cut off, without interrupting the patient in the sentence that he is uttering, is a surprising circumstance! From this fact Physiologists formerly inferred that the surgeon had not

* There are certain morbid conditions of sensation when cold bodies feel intensely hot.—*Dr. Abercrombie's Inquiry into the Intellectual powers.*

reached the more important organ of the brain. But that opinion arose from the notion prevailing that a nerve must necessarily be sensible. Whereas, when we consider that the different parts of the nervous system have totally distinct endowments, and that there are nerves, as I have elsewhere shewn, insensible to touch and incapable of giving pain, though exquisitely alive to their proper office, we have no just reason to conclude that the brain should be sensible, or exhibit the property of a nerve of the skin. Reason on it as we may, the fact is so ;—the brain, through which every impression must be conveyed before it is perceived, is itself insensible. This informs us that sensibility is not a necessary attendant on the delicate texture of a living part, but that it must have an appropriate organ, and that it is an especial provision.*

To satisfy my reader on this interesting subject, I shall take the contrast of two organs, one external and exposed, and the other internal and carefully excluded from injury.

The eye, consisting of its proper nerve of vision and its transparent humours and coats, is an organ of exquisite delicacy—not only is it exposed to all the injuries to which the general surface of the body is liable, but to be inflamed and rendered opaque by particles getting into it which are so light that they float in the atmosphere, and to the contact of which the common skin is quite insensible. The mechanical, and more obvious contrivance for the protection of this organ, is a ready motion of the eyelids and the shedding of tears ; which coming, as it were, from a little fountain, play over the surface of the eye, and wash away whatever is offensive. But to the action of this little hydraulic and mechanical apparatus there is required an exquisite sensibility to direct it—not that kind of sensibility which enables the eye to receive

---

* See the Sensibility of the Retina, Appendix.

the impressions of light—but a property more resembling the tenderness of the skin, yet happily adapted, by its fineness, to the condition of the organ.

A nerve, possessed of a quality totally different from that of the optic nerve, extends over all the exterior surfaces of the eye, and gives to those surfaces their delicate sensibility. Now it sometimes happens that this nerve is injured and its function lost; the consequences of which are very curious,—smoke and offensive particles, which are afloat in the atmosphere, rest upon the eye : flies and dust lodge under the eyelids, without producing sensation, and without exciting either the hydraulic or the mechanical apparatus to act for the purpose of expelling them. But although they do not give pain, they nevertheless stimulate the surfaces so as to produce inflammation, and that causes opacity in the fine transparent membranes of the eye ; and the organ is lost, although the *proper nerve of vision remains entire. I have seen many instances of the eye being thus destroyed for want of sensibility to touch,* and it has been curious to remark that when the hand was waved or a feather brought near the eye, the person winked ; yet he did not shut his eye on rubbing the finger across the eyeball, or when blood was removed by the lancet from the inflamed vessels. In those cases, when vision gave notice of danger to the organ, the patient winked to avoid it, but when the point touched the eye or eyelids, the sense of touch gave no alarm, and was followed by no action for the protection of the organ.

I shall present another instance of the peculiar nature of the sensibility which protects the eye. The Oculist has observed that by the touch of a thing as light as a feather, the muscles of the eye will be thrown into uncontrollable actions and spasms ; but if the point of the finger be pressed somewhat rudely

* They are stated at length in my papers in the Philosophical Transactions, and in the Appendix of my work on the Nervous System.

11*

between the eyelids, and directly on the eye itself, he can by such means hold the eye steady for his intended operation, producing hardly any sensation, certainly no pain !

This is one of the little secrets of the art; the Oculist turns out the eyelids, and fingers the eye, in a manner which appears, at once, rude and masterly : and still the wonder grows that he can do such things with so much dexterity as to inflict no pain, when by daily experience we know that even a grain of sand in the eye will torture us. The explanation is this : the eye and eyelids are possessed of a sensibility which is so adjusted as to excite the action of its protecting parts against such small particles as might lodge and inflame its fine membranes. But the apparatus is not capable of protecting the surface of the eye against the intrusion of a stick or a stone ; from such injuries it could not be defended by a delicate sensibility and involuntary action, but only by the effort of the will.

In these details we have new proofs of the minute relation which is established between the species of sensibility in an organ and the end to be attained through it. It will not be denied that but for the pain to which the eye is exposed, we should quickly lose the enjoyment of the sense of vision altogether. But we were about to institute a comparison of the eye with the heart.

The observation of the admirable Harvey, the discoverer of the circulation of the blood, is to this effect. A noble youth of the family of Montgomery, from a fall and consequent abscess on the side of the chest, had the interior marvellously exposed, so that after his cure, on his return from his travels, the heart and lungs were still visible and could be handled ; which when it was communicated to Charles I., he expressed a desire that Harvey should be permitted to see the youth and examine his heart. " When," says Harvey, " I had paid my respects to this young

" nobleman, and conveyed to him the king's request,
" he made no concealment, but exposed the left side
" of his breast, when I saw a cavity into which I
" could introduce my fingers and thumb; astonished
" with the novelty, again and again I explored the
" wound, and first marvelling at the extraordinary
" nature of the cure, I set about the examination of
" the heart.   Taking it in one hand, and placing the
" finger of the other on the pulse of the wrist, I
" satisfied myself that it was indeed the heart which
" I grasped.   I then brought him to the king that
" he might behold and touch so extraordinary a thing,
" and that he might perceive, as I did, that unless
" when we touched the outer skin, or when he saw
" our fingers in the cavity, this young nobleman
" knew not that we touched his heart !"   Other observations confirm this great authority, and the heart
is declared insensible.   And yet the opinions of mankind must not be lightly condemned.   Not only does
every emotion of the mind affect the heart, but every
change in the condition of the body is attended with
a corresponding change in the heart : motion during
health—the influence of disease—every passing
thought will influence it.   Here is the distinction
manifested.   The sensibility of the surface of the
eye is for a purpose, and so is the sensibility of the
heart.   Whilst that of the eye guards it against injury from without, the heart, insensible to touch, is
yet alive to every variation in the circulation, subject
to change from every alteration of posture or of
exertion, and is in sympathy of the strictest kind
with the constitutional powers.

When we consider these facts, we can no longer
doubt that the sensibilities of the living frame are appropriate endowments ; not qualities necessarily arising from life ; still less the consequences of delicacy
of texture.   Nor can we, I should hope, longer doubt
that they are suited to the condition, and especially
to the degree of exposure of each part, and for its pro-

tection. We perceive that the sensibilities vary in an extraordinary manner as they are given to external or to internal parts, as they belong to one apparatus of action or to another, and they are ever adapted to excite some salutary or necessary action. We perceive no instance of pain being bestowed as a source of suffering or punishment purely, or without finding it overbalanced by great and essential advantages—without, in short, being forced to admit that no happier contrivance could be found for the protection of the part. It is provided that the more an organ is exposed, and in proportion to its delicacy of organization—the more exquisitely contrived is the apparatus for its protection, and the more peremptory the call for the activity of that mechanism. The motive to action admits of no thought and no hesitation, and the action is more instantaneous than the quickest suggestion or impulse of the will.

We are speaking of the natural functions of the body. It requires a deeper consideration, and is indeed foreign to my subject to speak of the pains which result from disease, or to reconcile those who suffer in an extraordinary degree to the dispensations of Providence. But as a witness I may speak. It is my daily duty to visit certain wards of the hospital, where there is no patient admitted but with that complaint which most fills the imagination with the idea of insufferable pain and certain death. Yet these wards are not the least remarkable for the composure and cheerfulness of their inmates. The individual who suffers has a mysterious counterbalance to that condition, which to us who look upon her, appears to be attended with no alleviating circumstance.

It affords an instance of the boldness with which philosophers have questioned the ways of Providence, that they have asked—why were not all our actions performed at the suggestion of pleasure? why should we be subject to pain at all? In answer to this I should say, in the first place, that consistently with

our condition, our sensations and pleasures, there
must be variety in the impressions ; such contrast and
variety are common to every variety of sense ; and
the continuance of an impression on any one organ,
occasions it to fade. If the eye continue to look
steadfastly upon one object, the image is soon lost—
if we continue to look on one colour, we become insensible to that colour, and opposite colours to each
other are necessary for a perfect impression. So have
we seen that in the insensibilities of the skin variations are necessary to continued sensation.

It is difficult to say what these philosophers would
define as pleasure : but whatever exercise of the
senses it should be, unless we are to suppose an
entire change of our nature, its opposite is also
implied. Nay, further, in this fanciful condition of
existence, did anything of our present nature prevail,
emotions purely of pleasure would lead to indolence,
relaxation, and indifference. To what end should
there be an apparatus to protect the eye, since pleasure could never move us to its exercise? Could the
windpipe and the interior of the lungs be protected
by a pleasurable sensation attended with the slow
determination of the will—instead of the rapid and
powerful influence which the exquisite sensibility of
the throat has upon the act of respiration, or those
forcible yet regulated exertions, which nothing but
the instinctive apprehension of death could excite ?

To suppose that we could be moved by the solici-
tations of pleasure and have no experience of pain,
would be to place us where injuries would meet us
at every step and in every motion, and whether felt
or not, would be destructive to life. To suppose
that we are to move and act without experience of
resistance and of pain, is to suppose not only that
man's nature is changed, but the whole of exterior
nature also—there must be nothing to bruise the
body or hurt the eye, nothing noxious to be drawn in
with the breath : in short, it is to imagine altogether

another state of existence, and the philosopher would
be mortified were we to put this interpretation on his
meaning.   Pain is the necessary contrast to pleasure:
it ushers us into existence or consciousness : it alone
is capable of exciting the organs into activity : it is
the companion and the guardian of human life.

CHAPTER VIII.

OF THE SENSES GENERALLY, INTRODUCTORY TO THE SENSE OF TOUCH.

ALTHOUGH we are most familiar with the sensibility of the skin, and believe that we perfectly understand the nature of the impressions upon it and the mode of their conveyance to the sensorium, yet there is a difficulty in comprehending the operations of all the organs of the senses—a difficulty not removed by the apparent simplicity of that of touch.

There was a time when the enquirer was satisfied on finding that in the ear there was a little drum and a bone to play upon it, with an accompanying nerve. This was deemed a sufficient explanation of the organ of hearing. It was thought equally satisfactory if in experimenting upon the eye, the image was seen painted at the bottom of it on the surface of the nerve. But although the impression be thus traced to the extremity of the nerve, still we comprehend nothing of the nature of that impression, or of the manner in which it is transmitted to the sensorium. To the most minute examination, the nerves, in all their course, and where they are expanded into the external organs of sense, seem the same in substance and in structure. The disturbance of the extremity of the nerve, the vibrations upon it, or the images painted upon its surface, cannot be transmitted to the brain according to any physical laws that we are acquainted with. The impression on the nerve can have no resemblance to the ideas suggested in the mind. All that we can say is, that the agitations of the nerves of the outward senses are the

signals, which the Author of nature has made the
means of correspondence with the realities. There
is no more resemblance between the impressions on
the senses and the ideas excited by them, than there
is between the sound and the conception raised in
the mind of that man who, looking out on a dark and
stormy sea, hears the report of cannon, which conveys to him the idea of despair and shipwreck—or
between the impression of light on the eye, and the
idea of him who, having been long in terror of national convulsion, sees afar off a column of flame, which
is the signal of actual revolt.

By such illustrations, however, we rather show the
mind's independence of the organ of sense, and how
a tumult of ideas will be excited by an impression on
the retina, which, notwithstanding, may be no more
intense than that produced by a burning taper.
They are instances of excited imagination. But
even the determined relations which are established
in a common act of perception between the sensation
and the idea in the mind, have no more actual resemblance. How the consent, which is so precise and
constant, is established, can neither be explained by
anatomy nor by physiology, nor by any mode of physical inquiry whatever.

From this law of our nature, that certain ideas
originate in the mind in consequence of the operation
of corresponding nerves, it follows—that one organ
of sense can never become the substitute for another,
so as to excite in the mind the same idea.

When an individual is deprived of the organs of
sight, no power of attention, or continued effort of the
will, or exercise of the other senses, can make him
enjoy the class of sensations which is lost. The
sense of touch may be increased in an exquisite degree ; but were it true, as has been asserted, that individuals can discover colours by the touch, it could
only be by feeling a change upon the surface of the
stuff and not by any perception of the colour. It has

been my painful duty to attend on persons who have pretended blindness and that they could see with their fingers. But I have ever found that by a deviation from truth in the first instance, they have been entangled in a tissue of deceit; and have at last been forced into admissions which demonstrated their folly and weak inventions. I have had pity for such patients when they have been the subjects of nervous disorders which have produced extraordinary sensibility in their organs—such as a power of hearing much beyond our common experience; for it has attracted high interest and admiration, and has gradually led them to pretend to powers greater than they actually possessed. In such cases it is difficult to distinguish the symptoms of disease, from the pretended gifts which are boasted of.

Experiment proves, what is suggested by Anatomy, that not only the organs are appropriated to particular classes of sensations, but that the nerves, intermediate between the brain and the outward organs, are respectively capable of receiving no other sensations but such as are adapted to their particular organs.

Every impression on the nerve of the eye, or of the ear, or on the nerve of smelling, or of taste, excites only ideas of vision, of hearing, of smelling, or of tasting; not solely because the extremities of these nerves, individually, are suited to external impressions, but because the nerves are, through their whole course and wherever they are irritated, capable of exciting in the mind the idea to which they are appropriate, and no other. A blow, an impulse quite unlike that for which the organs of the senses are provided, will excite them all in their several ways; the eyes will flash fire, while there is noise in the ears. An officer received a musket-ball which went through the bones of his face—in describing his sensations, he said that he felt as if there had been a flash of lightning, accompanied with a sound like the shutting of the door of St. Paul's.

On this circumstance, of every nerve being appropriated to its function, depend the false sensations which accompany the morbid irritation of them from internal causes, when there is in reality nothing presented externally ;—such as flashes of light, ringing of the ears, and bitter taste or offensive smells. These sensations are caused, through the excitement of the respective nerves of sense, by derangement of some internal organ, and most frequently of the stomach.

But my chief object is to show that the most perfect proof of power and of design, is to be found in this, that the perceptions or ideas arising in the mind, are in correspondence with the qualities of external matter ; and that, although the manner in which the object presented to the outward sense and the idea of it are connected, must ever be beyond our comprehension, they are, notwithstanding, indissolubly united ; and when the object is so presented to us, it is attended with the conviction of its real existence—a conviction independent of reason and to be regarded as a first law of our nature.

The doctrine of vibrations acting on the nerve of vision, has had powerful advocates in our day. But it is quite at variance with anatomy, and assumes more than is usually granted to hypotheses. It requires that we shall imagine the existence of an ether ; and that this fluid shall have laws unlike anything of which we have experience. It supposes a nervous fluid and tubes of fibres in the nerve, to receive and convey these vibrations. It supposes everywhere *motion* as the sole means of propagating sensation.

These opinions have been formed on the misconception that if a certain kind or degree of vibration be communicated to any nerve, this particular motion must be propagated to the sensorium, and a corresponding idea excited in the mind. For example, it is conceived that if the nerve of hearing were placed in the bottom of the eye, it would be impressed with the vibration proper to light, and that this being conveyed to the brain, the sensation of light or colours would result—All which is contrary to fact.

Nor can I be satisfied that light and colours shall result from vibrations which shall vary "from four "hundred and fifty eight millions of millions, to "seven hundred and twenty seven millions of mil- "lions in a second," when I find that a fine needle pricking the retina will produce brilliant light, and that the pressure of the finger on the ball of the eye will give rise to all the colours of the rainbow!

There is a condition of the percipient or sentient principle, of the brain and nerves, as well as of the organ of sense, conforming to the impression to be made; a condition which corresponds with the qualities of matter. The several organs of sense may be compared to so many instruments, which the philosopher applies to distinguish the several qualities of the body which he investigates. The different properties of that body are not communicable through any one instrument; and so in the use of the senses, each organ is provided for receiving a particular influence, and no other.

However mortifying it may be to acknowledge ignorance, variation of motion in a body cannot be admitted as the cause of sensation universally; nor, as I said, can we comprehend anything of the manner in which the nerves are affected; certainly we know nothing of the manner in which sensation is propagated or the mind ultimately influenced. But there is a very pleasing view of the subject, notwithstanding; which is to observe the correspondence of the mind (through a series of organic parts) with the external world, or with the condition and qualities of matter: than which nothing can convey a more sublime idea of Power, and of the system or unity of organic and inorganic creations.

Returning to the consideration of the sensibility of

the skin and the sense of touch, this property is as distinct an endowment as that which belongs to the eye. It is neither inferior nor more common. It is not consequent upon the mere exposure of the delicate surface of the animal body. It is a distinct sense, the organ of which is seated in the skin ; and it is necessary that this organ of sense should be extended widely over the surface of the body. Yet the nerves are as appropriate and distinct as if they were gathered into one trunk, such as we find them to be in the organs of vision and hearing.

Although the portion of nervous matter on which the sensation and perception of touch depend, be necessarily extended in its sentient extremities over the whole exterior surface of the body, it is very much concentrated towards the brain : and it is there appropriated, in the same manner as the nerves of vision and of hearing, to its peculiar function of raising corresponding perceptions in the mind.

Perhaps this will be better understood from the fact—that a certain large portion of the skin may be the seat of excruciating pain, and yet the surface, which to the patient's perception is the seat of that pain, will be altogether insensible to cutting, burning, or any mode of destruction ! " I have no feeling in " all the side of my face, and it is dead ; yet surely " it cannot be dead, since there is a constant pricking " pain in it." Such were the words of a young woman whose disease was at the root of the nerve of sensibility near the brain.* The disease destroyed the function of this nerve of the head, as to its property of conveying sensation from the exterior : and substituted that morbid impression on the trunk which was referred to the tactile extremities.

If we use the term common sensibility, we can do so only in reference to touch, as it is the sense that is most necessary to animal existence, and as it is enjoyed by

* See Papers by the author in the Philosophical Transactions.

all animals from the lowest to the highest in the chain of existence.

While this sense is distinct from the others, it is the most important of all ; since through it alone some animals possess the consciousness of existence ; and to those that enjoy many organs of sense, that of touch, as we shall presently show, is necessary to the full developement of the powers of all the other organs.

OF THE ORGAN OF TOUCH.

Touch is that peculiar sensibility which gives the consciousness of the resistance of external matter, and makes us acquainted with the hardness, smoothness, roughness, size, and form of bodies. It enables us to distinguish what is external from what belongs to us ; and while it informs us of the geometrical qualities of bodies, we must refer to this sense also our judgment of distance, of motion, of number, and of time.

Presuming that the sense of touch is exercised by means of a complex apparatus—by a combination of the consciousness of the action of the muscles with the sensibility of the proper nerves of touch, we shall, in the first place, examine in what respect the organization resembles that of the other senses.

We have said before that, on the most minute examination of the extremity of a nerve, no appropriate structure can be detected ; and that the nerves expanded on the organs of sense appear every where the same,—soft, pulpy, prepared for impression, and so distributed that the impression shall reach them. What is termed the structure of the organs of sense, is that apparatus by which the external impression is conveyed inwards, and by which its force is concentrated on the extremity of the nerve. The mechanism by which those external organs are suited to their offices, is highly interesting ; it serves to shew (in a way that is level to our comprehension, as most resembling things of human contrivance) the design

with which the fabric is constructed.   Thus, the eye
is so seated and so formed as to embrace the greatest
possible field of vision.   We can understand the hap-
py effects of the convexity of the transparent cornea,
the influence of three humours of various densities acting like an achromatic telescope ; we can admire the
precision with which the rays of light are concentrated on the retina, and the beautiful provision for
enlarging or diminishing the pencil of light, in proportion to its intensity : but all this explains nothing, in
respect to the perception that is excited in the mind
by the impulse on the extremity of the nerve.

In like manner, in the complex apparatus of the
ear, we see how this organ is formed with reference
to a double course of impressions, as they come
through the solids or through the body, and as they
come through the atmosphere.   We comprehend how
the undulations and vibrations of the air are collected
and concentrated ; how they are directed, through
the intricate passages of the bone, to a fluid in which
the nerve of hearing is suspended ; and we see how,
at last, that nerve is moved.   But we can comprehend nothing more from the study of the external
organ of hearing.

The illustration is equally clear in reference to the
organ of smelling, or of taste.   There is nothing in
the nerve itself, either of the nose or of the tongue,
which can explain why it is susceptible of the particular impression.   For these reasons, we are prepared
to expect very little complexity in the organ of touch,
and to believe that the peculiarity of the sense consists more in the property bestowed on the nerve, than
in the mechanical adaptation of the exterior organ.

OF THE CUTICLE.

The cuticle or epidermis covers the true skin, ex-
cludes the air, limits the perspiration, and in some degree regulates the heat of the body.   It is a dead or

insensible covering ; it guards from contact the true vascular surface of the skin ; and in this manner, it often prevents the communication of infection. We are most familiar with it as that scarf skin which scales off after fevers, or by the use of the flesh-brush, or by the friction of the clothes ; for it is continually separating in thin scales, whilst it is as regularly formed anew by the vascular surface below. The condition of this covering is intimately connected with the organ of touch. The habit of considering things as produced accidentally, has induced some anatomists to believe that the cuticle is formed by the hardening of the true skin. The fact, however, that the cuticle is perfect in the new-born infant, and that even then it is thickest on the hands and feet, should have shewn that, like every thing in the animal structure, it participates in the great design.

The cuticle is the organ of touch in this respect, that it is the medium through which the external impression is conveyed to the nerves of touch ; and the manner in which this is accomplished is not without interest. The extremities of the fingers exhibit all the provisions for the exercise of this sense. The nails give support to the fingers ; they are formed broad and shield-like,* in order to sustain the elastic cushion which forms their extremity ; and the fulness and elasticity of the ends of the fingers adapt them admirably for touch. But on a nearer inspection, we see a more particular provision in the points of the fingers. Wherever the sense of feeling is most exquisite, there are minute spiral ridges of cuticle.— These ridges have, corresponding with them, depressed lines on the inner surface of the cuticle ; and these again give lodgement to a soft pulpy matter, in which lie the extremities of the sentient nerves. There the nerves are sufficiently protected, while they are exposed to impressions through the elastic cuticle,

* *Ungues scutiformis.*

and thus give the sense of touch. The organization is simple, yet it is in strict analogy with the other organs of sense.

Every one must have observed a tendency in the cuticle to become thickened and stronger by pressure and friction. If the pressure be partial and severe, the action of the true skin is too much excited, fluid is thrown out, and the cuticle is raised in a blister. If it be still partial, but more gradually applied, a corn is formed. If, however, the general surface of the palms or soles be exposed to pressure, the cuticle thickens, until it becomes a defence like a glove or a shoe. Now, what is most to be admired in this thickening of the cuticle is, that the sense of touch is not lost, or indeed diminished, certainly not at all in proportion to the protection afforded by the thickened skin.

The thickened cuticle partakes of the structure of the hoofs of animals: and we shall now attend to the nature of the hoof, as the best possible illustration of the manner in which the sensibility of the skin is in a due degree preserved whilst the surface is guarded.

The human nail is a continuation of the cuticle, and the hoof of an animal belongs to the same class of parts. In observing the manner in which the nerves enter the hoof, we have, in fact, a magnified view of that which exists, but is only more minute and delicate, in the fingers. We may take the horse's foot as the example. When the crust or hoof, which is insensible, is separated from the living part, we see small villi hanging from the vascular surface, and which have been withdrawn from the crust; looking to the inside of the crust, we perceive the pores from which these villi have been pulled. These processes of the living surface are not merely extremities of nerves; they consist of the nerves and the necessary accompaniments of membrane and bloodvessels, on a very minute scale. For it must be remembered that nerves can perform no function unless supplied with blood, all qualities of life being supported through the circulating blood. These nerves, so prolonged into the hoof, receive the vibrations of that body. By this means the horse is sensible to the motion and pressure of its foot, or to its percussion against the ground ; and without this provision, there would be a certain imperfection in the limb.

In a former part of this treatise I have shewn by what curious mechanism the horse's foot is made yielding and elastic, for the purpose of bearing the percussion against the ground. But in made roads, and with the imperfections of shoeing, the pressure and concussion are too severe and too incessant ; so that the protecting sensibility of the foot is converted into a source of pain from the inflammation which arises, and the horse is thus "foundered." There is a remedy for this condition in dividing the nerve ; the consequence of which operation is, that the horse, instead of moving with timid steps, puts out his feet freely, and the lameness is cured. If, however, we were to receive the statement thus barely, the fact would militate against our conclusion that mechanical provision and sensibility go together, being equally necessary to the perfection of the instrument. We must take into consideration this leading fact, that pressure against the sole and crust is necessary to the play of the foot and to its perfection. When this part becomes inflamed, the animal does not put its foot freely down, nor does it bear its weight upon the hoof so as to bring all the parts into action; hence contraction is produced, the most common defect of the horse's hoof. When the animal is relieved from pain by the division of the nerve, it uses the foot freely, and use restores all the natural actions of this fine piece of mechanism. It is obvious, however, that there is a certain defect ; the horse has lost his natural protection, and must now be indebted to the care of his rider. It has not only lost the pain which should guard against over exertion, but the feeling of the ground, which is necessary to his being perfectly safe as a roadster.

The teeth are provided with sensibility much in the same manner as the hoof of the horse is; for although the bone and enamel have no sensibility, yet a branch of a sensible nerve (the fifth) enters into the cavity of every tooth, and the vibration being communicated through the tooth to the nerve, the smallest grain is felt between the teeth.

But, to return to the human hand; in the fingers and palm of a man who uses the fore-hammer, the cuticle is thickened in a remarkable manner; the lines, however, become deeper, and the villi longer; which, joined to the aptitude of the cuticle to convey the impression to those included nerves, leaves him in possession of the sense of touch in a very high degree.

In the foot of the ostrich we may have a magnified view of the thickened cuticle and the lengthened nerves. The outer skin almost equals in thickness the hoof of the *solidungula*, and when it is separated from the sensible sole, the villi, or papillæ, having in them the sensible nerves, are withdrawn, leaving corresponding foramina or pores in the sole. We perceive that if the object had been merely to cover and protect the foot, it would have been sufficient to have invested it with a succession of solid and dead layers of cuticle. This would have been the case had the cuticle been merely thickened by pressure, and had there been no design to make a provision adapted in all respects to the habits of the bird.

Such, then, is the structure of the organ of touch: obvious in the extremities of the fingers; magnified in the foot of the horse or of the ostrich; and existing even in the delicate skin of the lips.

I have casually noticed that increased vascularity is always an accompaniment of nerves, and necessary to the sensibility of a part. In the museum of the College of Surgeons we see that Mr. Hunter had taken the pains to demonstrate this, by the injection of the bloodvessels of a slug. Although fluid was injected from its heart, the blush from the vermilion extends over its foot ; the foot, in these gasteropoda, being the whole lower flat surface on which the animal creeps. This surface is also the organ of touch, by which it feels and directs its motions. It is on the same principle, if we may compare such things, that we explain the rosy-tipped fingers and the ruby lips, which imply fine sensibility combined with high vascularity.

Having described the relation of the cuticle to the nerves of touch, we may take notice of another quality, in its roughness, and of the advantages accruing from this. In the first place, as to the subserviency of this quality to feeling, we must be sensible that in touching a finely polished surface the organ is but imperfectly exercised, as compared with its condition when we touch or grasp a rough and irregular body. Had the cuticle been finely polished on its surface it would have been but ill suited to touch: but, on the contrary, it has a very peculiar roughness which adapts it to feeling. A provision for friction, as opposed to smoothness, is a necessary quality of some parts of the skin. The roughness of the cuticle has the advantage of giving us a firmer grasp, and a steadier footing. Nothing is so little apt to slip as the thickened cuticle of the hand or foot. In the hoofs of animals, as might be expected, this structure is further developed. The chamois or goat steps securely on the ledges of rocks and at great heights, where it would seem impossible to cling. On the pads or cushions of the cat, the cuticle is rough and granular ; and in the foot of the squirrel, indeed of all animals which climb, those pads covered with the peculiar texture of the cuticle, give security in descending, as their claws enable them to climb.

In concluding this section, we perceive that the organ of touch consists of nerves appropriated to receive the impressions of bodies capable of affording resistance. Fine filaments of those nerves, wrapt up

in delicate membrane with their accompanying arteries and veins, project from the true skin into corresponding grooves or foramina of the cuticle.   They are
not absolutely in contact with the cuticle, but are
surrounded with a semi-fluid matter.   By this fluid
and by the cuticle they are protected, at the same
time that they are sensible to the pressure made on
the surface, and to cutting, pricking, and heat.*
But this capacity, we repeat, is not owing, strictly
speaking, to any thing in the structure of the organ,
but to the appropriation of the nerves to this class of
sensations.

* It is a curious confirmation of the fact, that the cutaneous nerve
is adapted to receive impressions from the varieties of temperature,
that when disease takes place in the centre of the trunk of a nerve,
or when the nerve is surrounded with diseased parts, the sensation of
burning accompanies the pain; and the patient refers this to the part
of the skin to which the extreme branch of the nerve is distributed.
By a burning sensation in the sole of the foot, I have been directed to
the disease seated in the centre of the thigh.

CHAPTER IX.

OF THE MUSCULAR SENSE.

Of the Sensibility of the Infant to Impressions, and the gradual improvement of the Sense of Touch.

A NOTION prevails that the young of animals are directed by instinct, but that there is an exception in regard to the human offspring : that in the child we have to trace the gradual dawn and progressive improvement of reason. This is not quite true ; we doubt whether the body would ever be exercised under the influence of reason alone, and if it were not first directed by sensibility which are innate or instinctive.

The sensibilities and the motions of the lips and tongue are perfect from the beginning : and the dread of falling is shewn in the young infant long before it can have had experience of violence of any kind.

The hand, which is to become the instrument for perfecting the other senses and developing the endowments of the mind itself, is in the infant absolutely powerless. Pain is poetically described as that power into whose " iron grasp" we are consigned, to be introduced to a material world ; now, although the infant is capable of an expression of pain, which cannot be misunderstood and is the same which accompanies all painful impressions during the whole life, yet it is unconscious of the part of the body which suffers. We have again recourse to the surgeon's experience. There occur certain congenital imperfections which require an operation at this early stage of life ; but the infant makes no direct effort with its hand to repel the instrument, or to disturb the dressing, as it will at a period somewhat later.

13

The lips and tongue are first exercised ; the next motion is to put the hand to the mouth, in order to suck it : and no sooner are the fingers capable of grasping, than whatever they hold is carried to the mouth. So that the sensibility to touch in the lips and tongue, and their motions, are the first inlets to knowledge ; and the use of the hand is a later acquirement.

The knowledge of external bodies as distinguished from ourselves, cannot be acquired until the organs of touch in the hand have become familiar with our own limbs ; we cannot be supposed capable of exploring any thing by the motion of the hand, or of judging of the form or tangible qualities of an object pressed against the skin, before we have a knowledge of our own body as distinguished from things external to us.

The first office of the hand, then, is to exercise the sensibility of the mouth : and the infant as certainly questions the reality of things by that test, as the dog does by its acute sense of smelling. In the infant, the sense of the lips and tongue is resigned only in favour of the sense of vision, when that sense has improved and offers a greater gratification, and a better means of judging of the qualities of bodies. The hand very slowly acquires the sense of touch, and many ineffectual efforts are seen in the arms and fingers of the child before the direction of objects or their distance is ascertained. Gradually the length of the arm, and the extent of its motions become the measure of distance, of form, of relation, and perhaps of time.

Next in importance to the sensibility of the mouth, we may contemplate that sense which is early exhibited in the infant,—the terror of falling. The nurse will tell us that the infant lies composed while she carries it in her arms up stairs ; but that it is agitated in carrying it down. If an infant be laid upon the arms and dandled up and down, its body and limbs will be at rest, whilst it is raised ; but they will struggle and make an effort as it descends. There is here the indication of a sense, an innate feeling of danger, the influence of which we may perceive when the child first attempts to stand or run. When the child is set upon its feet, and the nurse's arms form a hoop around it without touching it, it slowly learns to balance itself and stand; but under a considerable apprehension. Presently, it will stand at such a distance from the nurse's knee, that if it should lose its balance, it can throw itself for protection into her lap. In these its first attempts to use its muscular frame, it is directed by an apprehension which cannot as yet be attributed to experience. By degrees it acquires the knowledge of the measure of its arm, the relative distance to which it can reach, and the power of its muscles. Children, therefore, are cowardly by instinct: they show an apprehension of falling; and we may gradually trace the efforts which they make, under the guidance of this sensibility, to perfect the muscular sense. In the mean time, we perceive how instinct and reason are combined in early infancy: how necessary the first is to existence; how it is subservient to reason: and how it yields to the progress of reason, until it becomes so obscured that we can hardly discern its influence.

When treating of the senses, and showing how one organ profits by the exercise of the other, and how each is indebted to that of touch, I was led to observe that the sensibility of the skin is the most dependant of all on the exercise of another quality. Without a sense of muscular action or a consciousness of the degree of effort made, the proper sense of touch could hardly be an inlet to knowledge at all. I am now to show that the motion of the hand and fingers, and the sense or consciousness of their action, must be combined with the sense of touch, properly so called, before we can ascribe to it the influence which it possesses over the other organs.

In my general course of lectures on anatomy, I

ventured on this explanation from the commencement; much doubting, however, the correctness of
my reasoning, from seeing that the great authorities
on this subject made no account of the knowledge
derived from the motions of our own frame. I called
this consciousness of muscular exertion a sixth sense;
considering it as essential to the exercise of the sense
of touch. I can now refer, in confirmation of this
view, to the works of philosophers who have been
educated to medicine; and to whom the necessity of
the combination of the two faculties had suggested
itself as it had to me.*   Those distinctions were connected with my enquiries into the functions of the
nervous system, and in some measure directed
them.†

The Abbé Nollet, after extolling the sense of touch
as superior to all the other senses, and as deserving

* See Dr. Brown's Lectures on Moral Philosophy.

† It was this conviction—that we are sensible of the action of the
muscles, which led me to the investigation of their nerves; first, by
anatomy, and then by experiment. I was finally enabled to show
that the muscles had two classes of nerves—that on exciting one of
these, the muscle contracted; that on exciting the other, no action
took place. The nerve which had no power was found to be a nerve
of sensation: and thus, it was proved that there is a nervous circle
connecting the muscles with the brain: that one nerve is not capable
of transmitting what is called the nervous spirits, in two different
directions at one instant of time; but that for the regulation of the
muscles, there is a nerve of sensibility to convey the nervous influence
from the muscles towards the sensorium, as well as a nerve of action
for conveying the mandate of the will to the muscles. In their distribution through the body, the nerves which possess these two distinct powers are wrapped up, or, as it were, woven together in the
same sheath; and they present to the eye the appearance of one
nerve. It was only by examining the nerves at their roots, that is,
where they arise from different tracts of the brain and spinal marrow, and before they have coalesced, that I succeeded in demonstrat-
ing their distinct functions. In the face, the nerve of motion passes
by a circuitous course, apart from the nerve of sensation, to be distributed in the muscles; and therefore the distinct characters of these
nerves were more easily proved by experiment than in any other
part of the body. See the Philosophical Transactions on the "Nervous Circle which connects the Voluntary Muscles with the Brain,"
and the "Nervous System." 4to. Longman.

to be considered the *genus* under which the others should be included as subordinate *species*, makes this remark—" Besides, it has this advantage over them, " to be at the same time both active and passive ; for it " not only puts it in our power to judge of what makes " an impression upon us, but likewise of what resists " our impulsions." The mistake here lies in giving to the nerves of touch a property which must belong to the actions of muscles. So it is affirmed by physiologists, as I have already had occasion to state, that the sense of touch differs from the other senses by this circumstance—that an effort is propagated towards it, as well as a sensation received from it. This confusion obviously arises from considering the muscular agency, which is directed by the will during the exercise of touch, as belonging to the nerve of touch properly. We proceed to show how the sense of motion and that of touch are necessarily combined.

When a blind man, or a man with his eyes shut, stands upright, neither leaning upon, nor touching aught ; by what means is it that he maintains the erect position ? The symmetry of his body is not the cause ; the statue of the finest proportion must be soldered to its pedestal, or the wind will cast it down. How is it, then, that a man sustains the perpendicular posture, or inclines in due degree towards the winds that blow upon him ? It is obvious that he has a sense by which he knows the inclination of his body, and that he has a ready aptitude to adjust it, and to correct any deviation from the perpendicular. What sense then is this ? for he touches nothing, and sees nothing ; there is no organ of sense hitherto observed which can serve him, or in any degree aid him. Is it not that sense which is exhibited so early in the infant, in the fear of falling ? Is it not the full developement of that property which was early shown in the struggle of the infant while it yet lay in the nurse's arms ? It can only be by the adjustment of

13*

muscles that the limbs are stiffened, the body firmly balanced and kept erect. There is no other source of knowledge, but a sense of the degree of exertion in his muscular frame, by which a man can know the position of his body and limbs, while he has no point of vision to direct his efforts, or the contact of any external body. In truth, we stand by so fine an exer-. cise of this power, and the muscles are, from habit, directed with so much precision and with an effort so slight, that we do not know how we stand. But if we attempt to walk on a narrow ledge, or stand in a situation where we are in danger of falling, or rest on one foot, we become then subject to apprehension: the actions of the muscles are, as it were, magnified and demonstrative of the degree in which they are excited.

We are sensible óf the position of our limbs; we know that the arms hang by the sides; or that they are raised and held out; although we touch nothing and see nothing. It must be a property internal to the frame by which we know this position of the members of our body: and what can this be but a consciousness of the degree of action and the adjustment of the muscles? At one time, I entertained a doubt whether this proceeded from a knowledge of the condition of the muscles or from a consciousness of the degree of effort which was directed to them in volition. It was with a view to elucidate this, that I made the observations which terminated in the discovery that every muscle had two nerves—one for sensation, and one to convey the mandate of the will and direct its action. I had reasoned in this manner— we awake with a knowledge of the position of our limbs: this cannot be from a recollection of the action which placed them where they are; it must, therefore, be a consciousness of their present condition. When a person in these circumstances moves, he has a determined object; and he must be conscious of a previous condition before he can desire a change or direct a movement.

After a limb has been removed by the surgeon, the person still feels pain, and heat, and cold in it. Urging a patient to remove who has lost his limb, I have seen him catch at the limb to guard it, forgetful that it was removed ; and long after his loss, he experiences a sensation not only as if the limb remained, but as if it were placed or hanging in a particular position or posture. I have asked a patient—"Where do you feel your arm now?" and he has said, "I feel it "as if it lay across my breast," or that it is "lying "by my side." It seems also to change with the change of posture of the body. These are additional proofs of a muscular sense ; that there is an internal sensibility corresponding with the changing condition of the muscles; and that as the sensations of an organ of sense remain after the ' destruction of the outward organ, so here a deceptious sensibility to the condition of the muscles, as well as to the condition of the skin, is felt after the removal of the limb.

By such arguments I have been in the habit of showing that we possess a muscular sense, and that without it we could have no guidance of the frame. We could not command our muscles in standing, far less in walking, leaping, or running, had we not a perception of the condition of the muscles previous to the exercise of the will. And as for the hand, it is not more the freedom of its action which constitutes its perfection, than the knowledge which we have of these motions, and our consequent ability to direct it with the utmost precision.

The necessity for the combination of two distinct properties of the nervous system in the sense of touch becomes more obvious if we examine their operation in another but analogous organ ; for example, in the palpa or tentacula of the lower animals. These animals use those instruments to grope their way : and they consist of a rigid tube containing a pulpy matter, in which there is a branch of nerve that possesses in an exquisite degree the sense of touch. Now when this instrument touches a body and the vibration runs along the pulp of the nerve, the animal can be sensible only of an obstruction ; but where is that obstruction, and how is the creature's progress to be directed to avoid it ? We must acknowledge that the instrument moves about and feels on all sides, and that it is the action of the muscles moving this projecting instrument, and the sense of their activity, which convey the knowledge of the place or direction of the obstructing body.   It appears, therefore, that even in the very lowest creatures the sense of touch implies the comparison of two distinct senses.

That insects have the most exquisite organs of sense must be allowed : but we do not reflect on the extraordinary accuracy with which they measure distance ; which is an adaptation of the muscular exertion to the sense of vision.   The spider which I have already alluded to in a former chapter—the *aranea scenica*, when about to leap, elevates itself upon its fore legs, and lifting its head, seems to survey the spot before it jumps.   When this insect spies a small gnat or fly upon the wall, it creeps very gently towards it, with short steps, till it comes within a proper distance, and then it springs suddenly like a tiger. It will jump two feet to seize upon a bee.[*]

We have a more curious instance of the precision of eye and the adaptation of muscular action in the *chœtodon rostratus*.[†]   This fish inhabits the Indian rivers, and lives on the smaller aquatic flies.   When it observes a fly alighted on a twig or flying near (for it can shoot them on the wing) it darts a drop of water with so steady an aim as to bring the fly down into the water, when it falls an easy prey.   These fishes are kept in large vases for amusement, and if a fly be presented on the end of a twig, they will shoot at it with surprising accuracy.   In its natural state it will hit a fly at the distance of from three to

* Kirby.   † Chœtodon, a genus of the Acanthopterygii.

six feet. The *zeus insidiator** has also the power of
forming its mouth into a tube and squirting at flies so
as to encumber their wings and bring them to the
surface of the water. Whether led to admire the
wonderful power of instinct in these inferior creatures, or the property acquired by our own eye, we
must acknowledge a compound operation.†

The impression of odours on the nerve of smelling
is exactly what some would have us to believe the
effect of light is on the nerve of vision ; and yet,
that impression on the nerve of vision is sufficient, in
their opinion, to inform us of all that we know
through the eye. Now of the direction and distance
from which odours come, we are quite ignorant, until
by turning the head and directing the nostrils, and
moving this way and that, we make comparison, and
discover on which side the smell is strongest on the
sense. We can judge of the direction of sounds
without turning the head, because the strength of
vibration is unequal on the two sides of the head, and
a comparison is made of the two impressions. But
when a person is deaf of one ear the operation is
difficult ; he is often mistaken as to the direction of
sounds, and he has more necessity to turn the head
and to compare the position of the tube of the ear
with the strength of the impressions. Accordingly,
in mixed company, where there are many speakers,
he appears positively deaf, from the impossibility of
distinguishing minutely the direction of sounds.

The last proof of the necessity of the combination
of the muscular sense with the sense of contact will
be conclusive. The following is not a solitary instance :—

A mother while nursing her infant was seized with

* Belonging to another genus of the same Order.
† In these instances a difficulty will readily occur to the reader;
how does the fish judge of position, since the rays of light are refract-
ed at the surface of the water? Does instinct enable it to do this,
or is it by experience?

a paralysis, attended by the loss of power on one side of her body, and the loss of sensibility on the other side. The surprising, and, indeed, the alarming circumstance here was, that she could hold her child to her bosom with the arm which possessed muscular power, but only as long as she looked at the infant. If surrounding objects withdrew her attention from the state of her arm, the flexor muscles gradually relaxed and the child was in danger of falling. The details of the case do not belong to our present enquiry; but we see here, first, that there are two properties in the arm; which is shown by the loss of the one and the continuance of the other; secondly, that these properties exist through different conditions of the nervous system; and, thirdly, we perceive how ineffectual to the exercise of the limbs is the continuance of the muscular power, without the sensibility which should accompany and direct it.

The property in the hand of ascertaining the distance, the size, the weight, the form, the hardness and softness, the roughness or smoothness of objects results from the combined perception—through the sensibility of the proper organ of touch and the motion of the arm, hand, and fingers. But the motion of the fingers is especially necessary to the sense of touch; they bend, extend, or expand, moving in all directions like palpi, with the advantage of embracing the object, and feeling it on all its surfaces; sensible to its solidity and to its resistance when grasped; moving round it and gliding over its surface, and, therefore, feeling every asperity.

THE PLEASURES ARISING FROM THE MUSCULAR SENSE.

The exercise of the muscular frame is the source of much of the knowledge which is usually supposed to be obtained through the organs of sense; and to this source, also, we must trace some of our chief enjoyments. We may, indeed, affirm that it is benevolently provided that vigorous circulation, and, therefore, the healthful condition both of the mind and the body, shall result from muscular exertion and the alternation of activity and repose.

The pleasure which arises from the activity of the body is also attended by gratification from the exercise of a species of power—as in mere dexterity, successful pursuit in the field, or the accomplishment of some work of art. This activity is followed by weariness and a desire for rest, and although unattended with any describable pleasure or local sensation, there is diffused through every part of the frame, after fatigue and whilst the active powers are sinking into repose, a feeling almost voluptuous. To this succeeds the impatience of rest, and thus we are urged to the alternations which are necessary to health, and invited on from stage to stage of our existence.

We owe other enjoyments to the muscular sense. It would appear that in modern times we know comparatively little of the pleasures arising from motion. The Greeks, and even the Romans, studied elegance of attitude and movement. Their apparel admitted of it, and their exercises and games must have led to it. Their dances were not the result of mere exuberance of spirits and activity; they studied harmony in the motion of the body and limbs, and majesty of gait. Their dances consisted more of the unfolding of the arms than of the play of the feet,—"Their arms sublime that floated on the air." The Pyrrhic dances were elegant movements, joined to the attitudes of combat, and performed in correct coincidence with the expression of the music. The spectators in their theatres must have had very different associations from ours, to account for the national enthusiasm arising from music and their rage excited by a mere error in the time.

This reminds us that the divisions in music in some degree belong to the muscular sense. A man will put down his staff in regulated time, and the sound of his steps will fall into a measure, in his common walk. A boy striking the railing in mere wantonness, will do it with a regular succession of blows. This disposition of the muscular frame to put itself into motion with an accordance to time is the source of much that is pleasing in music, and aids the effect of melody. There is thus established the closest connection between the enjoyments of the sense of hearing and the exercise of the muscular sense.*

* To learn how much the enjoyment of the sense of vision belongs to motion, see the " Additional Illustrations," at the end of the volume.

CHAPTER X.

THE HAND NOT THE SOURCE OF INGENUITY OR CONTRIVANCE, NOR CONSEQUENTLY OF MAN'S SUPERIORITY.

SEEING the perfection of the hand, we can hardly be surprised that some philosophers should have entertained the opinion with Anaxagoras, that the superiority of man is owing to his hand. We have seen that the system of bones, muscles, and nerves of this extremity is suited to every form and condition of vertebrated animals ; and we must confess that it is in the human hand that we have the consummation of all perfection as an instrument. This, we perceive, consists in its power, which is a combination of strength with variety and extent of motion ; we see it in the forms, relations, and sensibility of the fingers and thumb; in the provisions for holding, pulling, spinning, weaving, and constructing ; properties which may be found in other animals, but which are combined to form this more perfect instrument.

In these provisions the instrument corresponds with the superior mental capacities, the hand being capable of executing whatever man's ingenuity suggests. Nevertheless, the possession of the ready instrument is not the cause of the superiority of man, nor is its aptness the measure of his attainments. So that we rather say with Galen—that man had hands given to him because he was the wisest creature, than ascribe his superiority and knowledge to the use of his hands.*

---

* Ita quidem sapientissimum animalium est homo ; ita autem et manus sunt organa sapienti animali convenientia. Non enim quia

14

This question has arisen from observing the perfect correspondence between the propensities of animals and their forms and outward organization. When we see a heron standing by the water side, still as a grey stone, and hardly distinguishable from it, we may ascribe this habit to the acquired use of its feet, constructed for wading, and to its long bill and flexible neck; for the neck and bill are as much suited to its wants as the lister is to the fisherman. But there is nothing in the configuration of the black bear particularly adapted to catch fish; yet he will sit on his hinder extremities by the side of a stream, in the morning or evening, like a practised fisher; there he will watch, so motionless as to deceive the eye of the Indian, who mistakes him for the burnt trunk of a tree; and with his fore paw he will seize a fish with incredible celerity. The exterior organ is not, in this instance, the cause of the habit or of the propensity; and if we see the animal in possession of the instinct without the appropriate organ, we can the more readily believe that, in other examples, the habit exists with the instrument, although not through it.

The canine teeth are not given without the carnivorous appetite, nor is the necessity of living by carnage joined to a timid disposition; but boldness and fierceness, as well as cunning, belong to the animal with retractile claws and sharp teeth, and which prey on living animals.*   On the other hand, the timid vegetable feeder has not his propensities produced by

---

manus habuit propterea est sapientissimum, ut Anaxagoras dicebat: sed quia sapientissimum erat, propter hoc manus habuit, ut rectissime censuit Aristoteles.   Non enim manus ipsæ homines artes docuerunt, sed ratio.   Manus autem ipsæ sunt artium organa: sicut lyra, musici, et forceps, fabri.

* In some of the quadrumana, the canine teeth are as long and sharp as those of the tiger—but they are in them only instruments of defence, and have no relation to the appetite, or mode of digestion, or internal organization.

the erect ears and prominent eyes ; though his disposition corresponds with them in his suspiciousness and timidity. The boldness of the bison or buffalo may be as great as that of the lion ; but the impulse is different—there is a direction given to him by instinct to strike with his horns : and he will so push whether he has horns or not. " The young calf will "butt against you before he has horns," says Galen : and the Scotch song has it " the putting cow is ay a doddy," that is, the humble cow (*inermis*), although wanting horns, is always the most mischievous. When that noble animal, the Brahmin bull, of the Zoological Gardens, first put his hoof on the sod and smelt the fresh grass after his voyage,—placid and easily managed before, he became excited, plunged, and struck his horns into the earth, and ploughed up the ground on alternate sides, with a very remarkable precision. This was his dangerous play ; just as the dog, in his gambols, worries and fights : or the cat, though pleased, puts out its claws. It would, indeed, be strange, where all else is perfect, if the instinctive character or disposition of the animal were at variance with its arms or instruments.

But the idea may still be entertained that the accidental use of the organ may conduce to its more frequent exercise and to the production of a corresponding disposition. Such an hypothesis would not explain the facts. The late Sir Joseph Banks, in his evening conversations, told us that he had seen, what many perhaps have seen, a chicken catch at a fly whilst the shell stuck to its tail. Sir Humphry Davy relates that a friend of his having discovered under the burning sand of Ceylon, the eggs of the alligator, he had the curiosity to break one of them ; when a young alligator came forth, perfect in its motions and in its passions ; for although hatched under the influence of the sunbeams in the burning sand, it made towards the water, its proper element : when hindered, it assumed a threatening aspect and bit the stick presented to it. As propensities to certain motions are implanted in animals, to which their external organs are subservient, so are passions given as the means of defence or of obtaining food. But this has been well said seventeen hundred years ago. "Take," says Galen, "three eggs, one of an eagle, another "of a goose, and a third of a viper; and place them "favourably for hatching. When the shells are "broken, the eaglet and the gosling will attempt to "fly; while the young of the viper will coil and twist "along the ground. If the experiment be protracted "to a later period, the eagle will soar to the highest "regions of the air, the goose betake itself to the "marshy pool, and the viper will bury itself in the "ground."

When we direct the enquiry to the comparison of man's faculties with his outward organization, the subject has increased interest. With the possession of an instrument like the hand there must be a great part of the organization, which strictly belongs to it, concealed. The hand is not a thing appended, or put on, like an additional movement in a watch; but a thousand intricate relations must be established throughout the body in connection with it—such as nerves of motion and nerves of sensation: and there must be an original part of the composition of the brain, which shall have relation to these new parts, before they can be put in activity. But even with all this superadded organization the hand would lie inactive, unless there were created a propensity to put it into operation.

I have been asked by men of the first education and talents whether any thing really deficient had been discovered in the organs of the orang-outang to prevent him from speaking! The reader will give me leave to place this matter correctly before him. In speaking, there is first required a certain force of expired air, or an action of the muscles of respiration; in the second place, the vocal chords in the top of the wind-pipe must be drawn into accordance by their muscles, else no vibration will take place, and no sound issue; thirdly, the open passages of the throat must be expanded, contracted, or extended by their numerous muscles, in correspondence with the condition of the vocal chords or glottis; and these must all sympathise before even a simple sound is produced. But to articulate that sound, so that it may become a part of a conventional language, there must be added an action of the pharynx, of the palate, of the tongue and lips. The exquisite organization for all this is not visible in the organs of the voice, as they are called: it is to be found in the nerves which combine all these various parts in one simultaneous act. The meshes of the spider's web, or the cordage of a man-of-war, are few and simple compared with the concealed filaments of nerves which move these parts; and if but one be wanting, or its tone or action disturbed in the slightest degree, every body knows how a man will stand with his mouth open, twisting his tongue and lips in vain attempts to utter a word.

It will now appear that there must be distinct lines of association suited to the organs of voice—different to combine them in the bark of a dog, in the neighing of a horse, or in the shrill whistle of the ape. That there are wide distinctions in the structure of the different classes of animals is most certain; but independently of those which are apparent, there are secret and minute varieties in the associating cords. The ape, therefore, does not articulate—First, because the organs are not perfect to this end. Secondly, because the nerves do not associate these organs in that variety of action which is necessary to speech. And, lastly, were all the exterior apparatus perfect, there is no impulse to that act of speaking.

Now I hope it appears, from this numeration of parts, that the main difference lies in the internal faculty or propensity. As soon as a child can distin-

14*

guish and admire, then are its features in action ; its voice begins to be modified into a variety of sounds ; these are taken up and repeated by the nurse, and already a sort of convention is established between them. We cannot, therefore, doubt that a propensity is created in correspondence with the outward organs, and without which they would be useless appendages. The aptness of the instrument or external organ will undoubtedly improve the faculty, just as we find that giving freedom to the expression of passion adds force to the emotion in the mind.

One cannot but reflect here on that grand revolution which took place when language, till then limited to its proper organ, had its representation in the work of the hand. Now that a man of mean estate can have a library of more intrinsic value than that of Cicero, when the sentiments of past ages are as familiar as those of the present, and the knowledge of different empires is transmitted and common to all, we cannot expect to have our sages followed, as of old, by their five thousand scholars. Nations will not now record their acts by building pyramids, nor consecrate temples and raise statues, once the only means of perpetuating great deeds or extraordinary virtues. It is in vain that our artists complain that patronage is withheld : for the ingenuity of the hand has at length subdued the arts of design—printing has made all other records barbarous, and great men build for themselves a " livelong monument."

Buffon has attempted to convey to us the mode in which knowledge may have been acquired by watching (in fancy) the newly awakened senses in the first created Man ; but, for that which is consistent and splendid in our great poet—who makes him raise his wondering eyes to Heaven and spring up by quick instinctive motion as " thitherward endeavouring," he substitutes a bad combination of philosophy with eloquence.

HAS MADE A REVOLUTION IN THE ARTS. 163

"To place the subject more distinctly before us,"
says Buffon, "the first created man shall speak for
"himself;" and the sentence which he is made to utter
is to the effect,—"that he remembers the moment
"of his creation—that time, so full of joy and trouble,
"when he first looked round on the verdant lawns and
"crystal fountains, and saw the vault of Heaven over
"his head;"—and he proceeds to declare,—"that he
"knew not what he was or whence he came, and be-
"lieved that all he saw was part of himself." He is
thus represented to be conscious of objects, which
even to see implies experience, and to enjoy, supposes a thousand disagreeable associations already
formed :—but from this blissful state he is awakened
by striking his head against a palm tree, which he
had not yet learned could hurt him !

Men are diffident of their first notions, and conceive that philosophy must lead to something very
different from what they have been early taught:
hence the absurdity of this combination of philosophy
and poetry. Later writers have argued that we have
no right to suppose that there has been, at any time,
an interruption to the course of nature. What they
term the uniformity of nature, is the prevalence of the
same laws which are now in operation. If, say they,
it happened that on the arrival of a colony in a new
country, fruits were produced spontaneously around
them, and flowers sprung up under their feet, then,
we might suppose that our first parents were placed
in a scene of beauty and profusion—suited to their
helpless condition—and unlike what we see now in
the course of nature.

It is not very wise to entertain the subject at all,
but if it is to be argued, this is starting altogether
wide of the question. We do not desire to know how a
tribe migrating westward could find sustenance, but
in what state man could be created to live without
a deviation from what is called the course of nature.

If man had been formed helpless as an infant, he

must have perished ; and if mature in body, he must
have been created with faculties suited to his condition.   A human being, pure from the Maker's hands,
with desires and passions implanted in him, adapted
to his state, and with a suitable theatre of existence,
implies something very near what we have been early taught to believe.

In every change which the globe has undergone,
we see an established relation between the animal
created, and the elements around it.   It is idle to suppose this a matter of chance.   Either the structure
and functions of the animal must have been formed
to correspond with the condition of the elements, or
the elements must have been controlled to minister
to the necessities of the animal ; and if the most careful investigation lead us to this conclusion, in contemplating all the inferior gradations of animal existence, what is it that makes us so unwilling to admit such an influence in the last grand work of
creation ?

We cannot resist those proofs of a beginning, or of
design prevailing everywhere, or of a First Cause.
When we are bold enough to extend our inquiries into the great revolutions which have taken place,
whether in the condition of the earth or in the structure of the animals which have inhabited it, our notions of the uniformity of the course of nature must
suffer some modification.   Changes must, at certain
epochs, have been wrought, and new beings brought
into existence different from the order of things previously existing, or now existing: and such interference
is not contrary to the great scheme of creation.   It is
not contrary to that scheme, but only to our present
state.   For the most wise and benevolent purposes, a
conviction is implanted in our nature that we should
rely on the course of events, as permanent and necessary.   We belong to a certain epoch ; and it is when
our ambitious thoughts carry us beyond our natural
condition, that we feel how much our faculties are

constrained, and our conceptions, as well as our language, imperfect. We must either abandon these speculations altogether, or cease to argue purely from our present situation.

It has been made manifest that man and the animals inhabiting the earth have been created with reference to the magnitude of the globe itself ;—that their living endowments bear a relation to their state of existence and to the elements around them. We have learnt that the system of animal bodies is simple and universal, notwithstanding the amazing diversity of forms that meet the eye—and that this system not only embraces all living creatures, but that it has been in operation at periods of great antiquity, before the last revolution of the earth's surface had been accomplished.

The most obvious appearances and the labours of the geologist give us reason to believe that the earth has not always been in the state in which it is now presented to us. Every substance which we see is compound ; we nowhere obtain the elements of things : the most solid materials of the globe are formed of decompounded and reunited parts. Changes have been wrought on the general surface, and the proofs of these changes are as distinct as the furrows on a field are indicative that the plough has passed over it. The deeper parts of the crust of the earth and the animal remains imbedded, also give proofs of revolutions : and that in the course of these revolutions there have been long periods or epochs. In short, progressive changes, from the lowest to the highest state of existence, of organization and of enjoyment, point to the great truth that there was a beginning.

When the geologist sees a succession of stratified rocks—the lowest simple, or perhaps chemical ; the strata above these, compound ; and successively others more conglomerated, or more distinctly composed of the fragments of the former—it is not easy to contradict the hypothesis of an eternal succession of causes. But there is nothing like this in the animal body, the material is the same in all, the general design too is the same: but each family, as it is created, is submitted to such new and fundamental arrangements in its construction as implies the presence of the hand of the Creator.

There is nothing in the inspection of the species of animals, which countenances the notion of a return of the world to any former condition. When we acknowledge that animals have been created in succession and with an increasing complexity of parts, we are not to be understood as admitting that there is here proof of a growing maturity of power, or an increasing effort in the Creator; and for this very plain reason, which we have stated, that the bestowing of life or the union of the vital principle with the material body, is the manifestation of a power superior to that displayed in the formation of an organ or the combination of many organs, or construction of the most complex mechanism. It is not, therefore, a greater power that we see in operation, but a power manifesting itself in the perfect and successive adaptation of one thing to another—of vitality and organization to inorganic matter.

In contemplating the chain of animal creation, we observe that even now, there are parts of the earth's surface which are marshy, and insalubrious, and that these are the places inhabited by amphibious and web-footed animals,—such as are suited to the oozy margins of swamps, lakes or estuaries. It is most interesting to find that when the remains of animals of similar construction, are found in the solid rocks, the geologist discovers by other signs that at the period of the formation of these rocks, the surface was flat, and that it produced such plants as imply a similar state of the earth to these swampy and unhealthy regions.

We mark changes in the earth's surface, and observe, at the same time, corresponding changes in the animal creation. We remark varieties in the outward form, size and general condition of animals, and corresponding varieties in the internal organization,—until we find men created of undoubted pre-eminence over all, and placed suitably in a bounteous condition of the earth.

Most certainly the original crust of the earth has been fractured and burst up, so as to expose its contents; that they might be resolved and washed away, by the vicissitudes of heat, cold, and rain. Mountains and valleys have been formed; the changes of temperature in the atmosphere have ensured continual motion and healthful circulation: the plains have been made salubrious, and the damps which hung on the low grounds have gathered on the mountains in clouds, so that refreshing showers have brought down the soil to fertilize the plain; thus at once have been supplied the means for man's existence, with objects suited to excite his ingenuity, and to reward it, and fitted to develope all the various properties both of his body and of his mind.

There is extreme grandeur in the thought of an anticipating or prospective intelligence: in reflecting that what was finally accomplished in man, was begun in times incalculably remote, and antecedent to the great revolutions which the earth's surface has undergone. Nor are these conclusions too vast to be drawn from the examination of a part so small as the bones of the hand; since we have shown that the same system of parts which constitutes the perfection of that instrument adapted to our condition, had its type in the members of those vast animals which inhabited the bays, and inland lakes of a former world. If we seek to discover the relations of things, how sublime is the relation established between that state of the earth's surface, which has resulted from a long succession of revolutions, and the final condition of its inhabitants as created in accordance with the change.

Nothing is more surprising to our measure of time.
than the slowness with which the designs of Providence have been fulfilled. But as far as we can
penetrate by the light of natural knowledge, the condition of the earth, and with it of man's destinies,
have hitherto been accomplished in great epochs.

We have been engaged in comparing the structure,
organs, and capacity of man and of animals—we
have traced a relation—but we have also observed a
broad line of separation : man alone capable of reason, affection, gratitude, and religion : sensible to
the progress of time, conscious of the decay of his
strength and faculties, of the loss of friends, and the
approach of death.

One who was the idol of his day has recorded
his feelings in nearly these words,—"We are as well
as those can be who have nothing further to hope or
fear in this world. We go in and out, but without
the sentiments that can create attachment to any
spot. We are in a state of quiet, but it is the tran-
quillity of the grave, in which all that could make
life interesting to us is laid." If in such a state there
were no refuge for the mind, then were there something wanting in the scheme of nature : an imperfection in man's condition at variance with the
benevolence which is manifested in all other parts of
animated nature.

ADDITIONAL ILLUSTRATIONS.

ADDITIONAL ILLUSTRATIONS.

THE MECHANICAL PROPERTIES OF THE SOLID STRUCTURE OF THE ANIMAL BODY CONSIDERED.

I YIELD to the suggestion of friends in further pursuing the subject of the solid textures of the animal frame, with the proofs of design which are exhibited in its mechanical provisions.

It has been shown in the first chapter that solidity and gravity are qualities necessary to every inhabitant of the earth : the first to protect it ; the second, that the animal may stand, and possess that resistance, which shall make the muscles available for action.

The first material to be taken notice of, which bestows this necessary firmness on the animal textures, is the *cellular substance.* This consists of delicate membranes, which form cells ; these cells communicate with each other, and the tissue thus composed enters every where into the structure of the animal frame. It constitutes the principal part of the *medusa,* which floats like a bubble on the water ; and it is found in every texture of the human body. It forms the most delicate coats of the eye, and gives toughness and firmness to the skin. It is twisted into ligaments, and knits the strongest bones : it is the medium between bone, muscle, and blood-vessel : it produces a certain firmness and union of the various component parts of the body while it admits of their easy motion. Without it, we should be rigid, notwithstanding the proper organs for motion ; and the cavities could not be distended or contracted, nor could the vessels pulsate.

But this cellular texture is not sufficient on all occasions, either for giving strength or protection : nor

does it serve to sustain the weight, unless the animal
live suspended in water, or creep upon the ground.
We see, therefore, the necessity for some harder and
more resisting material being added, if the weight is
to rest on points or extremities ; or if the muscular
activity is to be concentrated.

Nature has other means of supplying the fulcrum
and lever, besides the bones, or true skeleton, which
we have been examining in the first part of this volume : and perhaps we shall find that there may be a
system of solid parts superior to what we have been
studying in the *vertebrata.*

The larvæ of proper insects and the annelides have
no exterior members for walking or flying : but to
enable them to creep, they must have points of resistance, or their muscles would be useless.   Their
skins suffice ; they are hardened by a deposit within
them for this purpose ; but if this skin were not further provided, it would be rigid and unyielding, and
be no substitute for bone.   These hardened integuments are, therefore, divided into rings ; to these the
muscles are attached ; and as the cellular membrane
between the rings is pliant, these annelides can creep
and turn in every direction.

Without further argument, we perceive how the
skin, by having a hard matter deposited in it, is adapted to all the purposes of the skeleton.   It is worthy
of notice that some animals, still lower in the scale,—
the tubipores, sertularia, cellularia, &c., exhibit something like a skeleton.   They are contained within a
strong case from which they can extend themselves :
whilst the corals and madrepores, on the other hand,
have a central axis of hard material, the soft animal
substance being, in a manner, seated upon it.   But these
substitutes for the skeleton are, like shell, foreign to the
living animal ; although in office they may resemble
bone in sustaining the softer substance and giving form.

In the proper insect I should say that there is a
nearer approach to a skeleton, did it not appear that

the apparatus is more perfect than in some of the animals which have a true skeleton. The resisting material is here deposited externally, and is converted to every purpose which we have seen attained by means of the skeleton. Distinct members are formed, with the power of walking, leaping, flying, holding, spinning, and weaving. The hardened integuments, thus articulated and performing the office of bones, have, like them, spines and processes : with this difference, that their aspect is towards the centre, instead of projecting exteriorly. Were we to compare the system of " resisting parts" in man and in the insect, we should be forced to acknowledge the mechanical provisions to be superior in the lower animal ! The first advantage of the skeleton (as we may be permitted to call the system of hard parts in the insect) being external and lifeless, is, that it is capable of having greater hardness and strength bestowed upon it, according to the necessities of the animal, than can be bestowed upon bone : true bone being internal and growing with the animal, is penetrated with blood vessels ; and therefore must be porous and soft. The next advantage is mechanical. The hard material is strong to resist fracture, and to bear the action of muscles, in proportion to its distance from the centre : for the muscles in the insect, instead of surrounding the bones, as in the higher animals, are contained within the shell, and the shell is, consequently, so much the further thrown off from the axis.

When considering the larger vertebral animals, we had reason to say that there is a correspondence between the resistance of the bones and the power of the muscles, and we may indulge the same reflection here. As the integument covering the insect is much harder than bone, so are the muscles stronger, compared with the muscles of the vertebrata. From the time of Socrates, comparisons have been made between the strength of the horse and of the insect ; to the obvious superiority of the latter.

15*

As goodly a volume has been written on the muscles of a caterpillar as has ever been dedicated to the human myology. A very minute anatomical description has been made of the caterpillar which feeds upon the willow; and here we see that the annular construction of the hard integument determines the plan of the whole anatomy : the arrangement of the muscles, and the distribution of the nerves. Each ring has its three sets of muscles; direct, oblique, traversing and interweaving, but yet distinct and symmetrical; and all as capable of being minutely described as those of the human body have been by Albinus.* Corresponding with these muscles, the system of nerves is delicately laid down. In short, we allow ourselves to be misled in supposing that animals, either of minute size or low in the scale of arrangement, exhibit any neglect or imperfection. Even if they were more simple in structure, the admiration should be the greater : since they have all the functions in full operation which are necessary to life.

We may perceive that a certain substance calculated to sustain the more strictly living part, and to give strength, may be traced through all living bodies. In the vegetable it is the woody fibre ; and there, sometimes, as if to mark the analogy, we may find silicious earth deposited instead of the phosphate and carbonate of lime of the animal structure. In the lower animals we find membranes capable of secreting a solid material, and although in some instances the substance is like leather or cartilage, it is in general earthy, and for the most part, carbonate of lime. But when elasticity is necessary, as well as general resistance, cartilage is employed, which is a highly comprehensible and elastic substance. Thus, in fishes, there is a large proportion of cartilage in their bones, and from this greater quantity, some have

* The work referred to is by Lyonnet, who reckons four thousand and sixty one muscles in this caterpillar. He was, I think, a lawyer, with little to do.

been called cartilaginous in distinction to the osseous
or true fishes.   The cartilaginous and elastic skeleton is brought into use in an unexpected manner :
when the salmon or trout leaps from the water, the
muscles bend the elastic spine,—which recoils in aid
of the muscles of the opposite class : and thus these
two forces combine to give a powerful stroke with the
tail on the water.

MECHANICAL PROPERTIES IN BONE OR IN THE TRUE SKELETON.

These considerations lead us the more readily to
understand the composition of bone : which is a combination of three parts having different properties,—
membrane, phosphate of lime, and cartilage.   By
these it is enabled to resist stretching, compression,
and tortion.   If bone had a superabundance of the
earthy parts, it would break like a piece of porcelain ;
and if it did not possess toughness and some degree
of elasticity, it would not enable a man to pull and
push and twist.

Looking to the dense bone, we should hardly suppose that it was elastic ; but if ivory be possessed of
elasticity, it cannot be denied to bone.   Now if a bil-
liard ball be put upon a marble slab which has been
painted, a very small spot will mark where the contact has been ; but if we let the ball drop upon the
marble from a height, we shall find the spot much
larger, and that the elasticity of the ivory has permitted the ball to yield and momentarily to assume
an oblate spheroidal form.

When a new principle is admitted into a complex
fabric, the utmost ingenuity can hardly anticipate all
the results.   Elasticity is extensively employed in the
machinery of the animal body ; and to show how finely it must be apportioned, we shall take the instance
of a bridge built with iron instead of stone, and hav-

ing a certain swing and elasticity. It lately happened that a bridge of this kind fell in very curious circumstances,—by the marching of a body of soldiers over it. Now the bridge was calculated to sustain a greater weight than this body of men : and had they walked tumultuously over it, it would have withstood the pressure : but the soldiers marching to time, accumulated a motion, aided by the elasticity of the material, which broke it down. This leads us to form a conception of the necessity of the fine adjustment of the material in the animal fabric ; not merely to enable it to sustain the incumbent weight, or transverse or oblique impulses, but to withstand the frequent, and regularly repeated forces to which it may be subject in the various actions of the body. It gives interest to this fact, that there is hardly a bone but what has a constitution of its own, adjusted to its place and use : the heel bone, the shin bone, the vertebræ, and the bones of the head, differ in mechanical construction. But the consideration of these adaptations in the constitution of the bones makes some general remarks necessary.

Perfect security against accidents in the animal body, and in man especially, is not consistent with the scheme of nature. Without the precautions and the continued calls to exertion, for safety, which danger and the uncertainty of life produce, many of the faculties of the mind would remain unexercised ; and whence else would come courage, resolution, and all the manly virtues ? Take away the influence of the uncertain duration of life, and we must suppose also a change in the whole moral constitution of man. Whether we consider the bones as formed to protect the part, as in the skull : or to be levers to which the muscles are attached, as in the limbs : or in both capacities, as in the texture of the chest : while they are perfectly adapted to their function, they are yet subject to derangements from accident. The mechanical adaptations which we have to observe are perfectly sufficient to their ends, and afford safety in the natural exercises of the body. To these exercises there is an intuitive impulse, ordered with a relation to the frame of the body; whilst, on the other hand, we are deterred from the excessive or dangerous use of the limbs by the admonitions of pain. Without such considerations, the reader would fall into the mistake that weakness and liability to fracture implied imperfection in the frame of the body: whereas a deeper contemplation of the subject will convince him of the incomparable perfection both of the plan and of the execution. The body is intended to be subject to derangement and accident, and to become, in the course of life, more and more fragile, until by some failure in the frame-work or vital actions, life terminates.

The bones of the extremities are called hollow cylinders. Now, after we have convinced ourselves of the necessity of this formation, we find these bones, upon a more particular examination, extremely varied in their shapes: and we are, at last, prone to believe that there is much of chance or irregularity in their shapes; but such a conception is quite inconsistent with a correct knowledge of the skeleton. As this notion, however, is very commonly entertained and leads to further mistakes, we shall take pains to show,—first, why the bones are hollow; and, in the second place, why they vary in their shape, so as to appear to the superficial observer irregular.

The reasoning that applies to the hollow cylindrical bone serves equally to explain many other natural forms, as that of a quill, a reed, or a straw. The last example reminds us of the unfortunate man who was drawn from his cell before the Inquisition, and accused of having denied that there was a God; when picking up a straw that had stuck to his garments, he said, " If there were nothing else in nature to teach " me the existence of a Deity, this straw would be " sufficient." It hardly requires demonstration to

prove that, with a given mass of material to make a
pillar or column, the hollow cylinder will be the
form of strength.   The experiments of Du Hamel on
the strength of beams afford us the best illustration
how the material should be arranged to resist transverse fracture.   When a beam rests on its extremities,
bearing a weight upon its centre, it admits of being
divided into three portions ; for these three parts are
in a different condition with regard to the weight.
The lower part resists fracture by its toughness : the
upper part, by its density and resistance to compression : but there is a portion between these which is
not acted upon at all ; which might be taken away
without any considerable weakening of the beam :
and which might be added to the upper or the lower
part with great advantage.   It can readily be understood how a tougher substance added to the lower
part would strengthen the beam : we see it in the
skin which is laid along the back part of the Indian's
bow ; or in the leather of a carriage spring : but the
following is a beautiful experiment to demonstrate
that quality in the timber which resists, at the upper
portion of the beam.   If a portion amounting to
nearly a third part of the beam be cut away and a
harder piece of wood be nicely let into the space, the
strength will be increased ; because the hardness of
this piece of wood resists compression.   This experiment I like the better because it explains a very interesting peculiarity in the different densities of the
several parts or sides of the bones.   In reading anatomical books, we are led to the supposition that the
various forms of the bones result from the pressure of
the muscles.   This is a mistake.   Were we to consider this the true explanation, it would not only be
admitting an imperfection, but we should expect to
find, if the bones yielded in any degree to the force
of the muscles, that they would yield more and more,
and be ultimately destroyed.   There is nothing more
admirable in the living frame than the relation esta-

blished between the muscular power and the capacity
of passive resistance in the bones.   The deviations
from the cylindrical forms are not irregularities; and
if we take that bone which deviates the furthest from
the cylindrical shape, the tibia, or shin bone, we shall
have demonstration of the relation between the shape
of the bone and the force which it has to sustain.

If we consider the direction of the force in walking,
running, or leaping, and in all the powerful exertions
where the weight of the body is thrown forwards on
the ball of the great toe, it must appear that the pressure against this bone is chiefly on the anterior part :
and there is no doubt that if the tibia were a perfect
cylinder, it would be subject to fracture even with
the mere force of the body itself thrown upon it. . But
if, as we have stated, the column is stronger in proportion as the material is distant from the centre, we
readily perceive how an anterior spine or ridge, should
be thrown out : and if we attend to the internal structure of that spine, we shall find that it is much denser
and stronger than the rest of the bone.   We cannot
here deem either the form or the density of this ridge,
a thing of accident; since it so perfectly corresponds
with the experiment of Du Hamel which we have described, where the dense piece of wood being let into
the piece of timber, it was found to be a means of resisting transverse fracture. If we proceed with the knowledge of these facts to the examination of the different
bones of the skeleton, we shall find that every where
the form has a strict relation either to the motion to be
performed, or the strain to which the bone is liable.

In comparing the true bones with the coverings of
the insects, we observed the necessity for the porous
structure of the former.   If it be necessary that the
bone shall be very dense, it will no longer be possessed
of the power of re-union or reproduction when it
breaks : it will not re-unite upon being fractured, and
if exposed, it will die.   Here, then, is an obvious imperfection.   The bones of animals cannot, in this man-

ner, be made capable of sustaining great weight, without losing a property which is necessary to their existence—that of restoration on their being injured. And even were the material very much condensed, it does not appear that the phosphate of lime, united as it is with the animal matter, is capable of sustaining any great weight ; this accordingly limits the size of animals.   It may, perhaps, countenance the belief that animals bear a relation in their size and duration of life, to the powers and life of man, that the larger animals have existed in a former condition of the world.   We allude only to such animals as have extremities : for with respect to the whale, its huge bulk lies out supported on the water.   The iguanadon, discovered by Mr. Mantell, is estimated to have been seventy feet in length, and to have had extremities. But the thigh and leg did not exceed eight feet in length, while the foot extended to six feet ; a proportion, altogether, which implies that the extremities assisted the animal to crawl, rather than that they were capable of bearing its weight, as the extremities of the mammalia.   However, we find that in the larger terrestrial animals, the material of the bones is dense, and that their cavities are filled up : the diameters of those of the extremities, with their spines and processes being remarkably large.   Nothing can be conceived more clumsy than the bones of the megatherium : so that it really appears that nature has exhausted her resources with respect to this material ; and that living and vascular bone could not be moulded into a form to sustain the bulk and weight of an animal much superior to the elephant, mastodon, and megatherium.*

* The subject may be illustrated in this manner :—"A soft stone "projecting from a wall, may make a stile strong enough to bear a "person's weight; but if it were necessary to double the length of the "stile, the thickness must be more than doubled, or a freestone sub- "stituted; and were it necessary to make this freestone project twice "as far from the wall, even if doubled in thickness, it would not be

With regard to the articulation of the bones, we cannot mistake the reason of the surfaces of contact being enlarged. In machinery it is found that, if the pressure be the same, the extension of the surfaces in contact does not increase the friction. If, for example, a stone or a piece of timber, of the shape of a book or a brick, should be laid upon a flat surface, it would be drawn across it with equal facility, whether it rested upon its edge or upon its side. The friction of the bones· which enter into the knee joint is not increased by their greater diameter : while great advantages are gained ; the ligaments which knit these bones give more strength than they otherwise would, and the tendons which run over them, being removed to a distance from the centre, have more power.

THE MUSCULAR AND ELASTIC FORCES.

The muscular power is contrasted with the elastic, as possessing a living property of motion. We acquiesce in the distinction, since the muscular fibre ceases to have irritability or power in death, while elasticity continues in the dead part. But yet there is a property of elasticity in the living body which cannot be retained after death. To illustrate this we shall take the instance of the catgut string of a harp. Suppose that the string is screwed tight, so as to vibrate in a

" strong enough to bear a proportioned increase of weight : granite
" must be placed in its stead ; and even the granite would not be
" capable of sustaining four times the weight which the soft stone
·" bore in the first instance. In the same way the stones which form
" an arch, of a large span, must be of the hardest granite, or their
" own weight would crush them. The same principle is applicable
·" to the bones of animals. The material of bone is too soft to admit
" an indefinite increase of weight ; and it is another illustration of
" what was before stated, that there is a relation established through
" all nature : that the very animals which move upon the surface of
" the earth are proportioned *to its magnitude*, and the gravitation to
" its centre."—Animal Mechanics.

16

given time, and to sound the note correctly; if that string be struck rudely, it is put out of tune; that is, it is stretched and somewhat relaxed, and no longer vibrates in time. This does not take place in the living fibre: for here there is a property of restoration. If we see the tuner screwing up the harp string, and with difficulty, and after repeated attempts, bringing it to its due tension,—trying it with the tuning fork, and with his utmost acquired skill restoring it to its former elasticity, we have a demonstration of how much life is performing in the fibres of the animal frame, after every effort or exertion; and the more powerful the mechanical parts of the body are, the more carefully is the proper tension of the tendons, ligaments, and heart-cords preserved. Or we may take the example of a steel spring. A piece of steel, heated to a white heat, and plunged into cold water, acquires certain properties; and if heated again to 500 of Fahrenheit, it is very elastic; possessing what is called a "spring temper," so that it will recoil and vibrate. But if this spring be bent in a degree too much, it will lose part of its elasticity. Should the parts of the living body, on the other hand, be thus used, they have a power of restoration which the steel has not.

If a piece of fine mechanism be made perfect by the workman, it may be laid by and preserved; but it is very different with the animal body. The mechanical properties of the living frame, like the endowments of the mind, must not lie idle, or they will suffed deterioration. If, by some misfortune, a limb be put out of use, not only is the power of the muscles rapidly diminished, which every one will acknowledge, but the property of resistance is destroyed; and bones, and tendons, and ligaments quickly degenerate.*

* This subject is illustrated in the Essay on Animal Mechanics, Part II.

If we are in search of an object which shall excite the highest interest, and at the same time afford proofs of design in the most delicate of all the organs of the body, we naturally turn to the eye : and this organ suits our present purpose the better, that we have to show how much of the sense of vision depends on the hand, and how strict the analogy is between the two organs.

From the time of Sir Henry Wotton to the latest writer on light, the eye has been a subject of admiration and eulogy. But I have ventured, on a former occasion,* to say, that this admiration is misplaced, while it is given to the ball of the eye and the optic nerve exclusively ; since the high endowments of this organ belong to the exercise of the whole eye, to its exterior apparatus, as much as to its humours and the proper nerve of vision. It is to the muscular apparatus, and to the conclusions which we are enabled to draw from the consciousness of muscular effort, that we owe that sense by which we become familiar with the form, magnitude, and relations of objects. One might as well imagine that he understood the effect and uses of a theodolite, on estimating the optical powers of the glasses, without looking to the quadrant, level, or plumb-line, as suppose that he had learnt the whole powers of the eye by confining his study to the naked ball.

We must begin our observations by a minute attention to the structure and sensibility of the retina. The retina is the internal coat of the eye ; it consists of a delicate, pulpy, nervous matter, which is contained between two membranes of extreme fineness, and these membranes both support it and give to its

* See Philosophical Transactions.

surfaces a mathematical correctness.   The matter
of the nerve, as well as these supporting membranes,
are perfectly transparent, during life; and on the
axis of the eye, there is a small portion which remains
transparent, when the rest of the membrane becomes
opaque, and which has been mistaken for a foramen,*
or hole in the retina.   It is surprising, that with all
the industry which has been employed to demonstrate
the structure of the eye, it is only in the present day
that a most essential part of the retina has been discovered—the membrane of Mr. Jacob.   From observing the phenomena of vision, and especially the
extreme minuteness of the image cast upon the retina, I had conceived that the whole nerve was not the
seat of vision, but only one or other of its surfaces.
This could not be well illustrated until the exterior
membrane of the retina was demonstrated.   But
now we see that this membrane, when floated in
water and under a magnifying glass, is of extreme
tenuity, and its smooth surface is well calculated to
correspond with the exterior surface of that layer of
nervous matter which is the seat of the sense.

The term retina would imply that the nerve constitutes a net-work : and the expressions of some of
our first modern authorities would induce us to believe that they view it in this light, as corresponding
with their hypothesis.   But there is no fibrous texture in the matter of the nerve ; although, when the
retina is floated and torn with the point of a needle,
the innermost of the membranes which support the
nerve, the *tunica vasculosa retinæ*, presents something
of this appearance.

Vision is not excited by light unless the rays penetrate through the transparent retina and reach the
exterior surface from within.

It is well known, that if we press upon the eye-
ball with a key or the end of a pencil-case, zones of

---

* It is this part which is called the foramer of Soemmerring.

light are excited. The perception of that light is, as if the rays came in a direction opposite to the pressure. We may say that, in this case, the effect of the pressure is assimilated to that of light; and as light can strike the part of the nerve which is pressed, only by coming in an opposite direction, the zones of light produced by the mechanical impulse appear in the usual direction of rays impinging upon this part: and consequently, they give the impression of their source being in the opposite quarter. Let us contrast this phenomena with the following experiment. Close the eyelids, and cover them with a piece of black cloth or paper which has a small hole in it; and place this hole, not opposite to the pupil, but to the white of the eye; direct a beam of light upon the hole; a person will see this light in its true direction. Why should there be in these two cases a difference in the apparent place from which the light is derived? were it not that the rays of light directed upon the eye-ball, after striking upon the retina, pierce through it and through the humours of the eye, and impinge upon the retina on the opposite side. This explains why the light excited in the eye shall appear to come from different quarters; but it does not explain why there should not be a double impression—why the beam of light should not influence the retina while penetrating it in the first instance, that is in passing through it from without inwards, as well as when it has penetrated the humours and strikes upon the opposite part of the retina from within outwards.

Another fact, which has surprised philosophers, is the insensibility of the optic nerve itself to light. If it be so contrived that the strongest beam of light shall fall upon the end of the nerve at the bottom of the eye, where it begins to expand into the delicate retina, no sensation of light will be produced. This ought not to surprise us, if I am correct in my statement that the gross matter of the nerve is not the

16*

organ of vision, but the exterior surface of it only. In the extremity of the optic nerve there is, of course, no posterior surface; and, indeed, nothing can better prove the distinct office of the nerve as contrasted with the expanded retina, than this circumstance, that when the strongest ray of light strikes into the nerve itself, the impression is not received. It seems to imply, that the capacity of receiving the impression, and of conveying it to the sensorium, are two distinct functions.

Is not this opinion more consistent with the phenomena than what is expressed by one of our first philosophers, that the nerve, at its extremity towards the eye, forms what has been called the *punctum cœcum*, and is insensible, because it is not yet divided into those almost infinitely minute fibres which are fine enough to be thrown into tremors by the rays of light.

Independently of this punctum cœcum, we have to observe that the whole surface of the retina is not equally sensible to light. There is a small spot, opposite to the pupil and in the axis of the eye, which is more peculiarly sensible to visual impressions. An attempt has been made to ascertain the diameter of this spot; and it is said, that a ray at an angle of five degrees from the optic axis, strikes exterior to this sensible part. But we shall, on the contrary, see reason to conclude, that the sensible spot is not limited to an exact circle, that it is not regularly defined, and that the sensibility, in fact, is increasing to the very centre.

Some have denied the existence of this extreme sensibility in the centre of the retina, attributing the distinctness of the vision to the circumstance of the light being made to converge through the influence of the humours, more correctly to this point. I shall, therefore, show how impossible vision would be, were it not that the sensibility of the retina increases gradually from its utmost circumference to the point which forms the axis of the eye.

We see objects by reflected light, at the very instant that direct light enters the eye. As the impression by the direct light is many times stronger than the reflected rays from the object, the vision of the object would be destroyed by the contrast, were there not this admirable provision in the retina, that the direct light shall fall upon a part less sensible, the reflected light upon a part more sensible. If, in full day, and in the open field, the eye be directed southward, the rays from the sun enter the eye at the time that we are looking to certain objects. It is perfectly clear, that if the sun's rays struck a part of the retina as sensible as the spot in the centre or axis, it would extinguish all secondary impressions: the glare would be painfully powerful, as when we look directly to the sun. If a momentary glance to the sun produce a sensation so acute that we see nothing for some time after, would not the same happen were the retina equally sensible in all its surface? A similar thing takes place in a chamber lighted with candles; we do not see the person immediately on the other side of the candle: for there the direct light interferes with the reflected light, effacing the slighter impression of the latter.

We perceive, therefore, that if the retina were equally sensible over all its surface we could not see. Let us, then, observe how we do actually see, and how the organ is exercised. There is a continual desire of exercising the sensible spot, the proper seat of vision. When an impression is made upon the retina, in that unsatisfactory degree, which is the effect of its striking any part but the centre, there is an effort made to direct the axis towards it, or, in other words, to receive the rays from it upon the more sensible centre. It is this sensibility, therefore, conjoined with the action of the muscles of the eye-ball, which produce the constant searching motion of the eye; so that, in effect, from the lesser sensibility of the retina generally, arises the necessity for this exercise of the organ ; and to this may be attributed the high perfections of it.

This faculty of searching for the object is slowly acquired in the child : and, in truth, the motions of the eye are made perfect, like those of the hand by slow degrees. In both organs there is a compound operation :—the impression on the nerve of sense is accompanied with an effort of the will, to accommodate the muscular action to it. It is no contradiction to this, that the faculty of vision is made perfect in the young of some animals from the beginning ; no more than the instinct of the duck, when it runs to the water the moment that the shell is broken, contradicts the fact that the child learns to stand and walk after a thousand repeated efforts.

Let us now see how essential this searching motion of the eye is to vision. On coming into a room, we see the whole side of it at once—the mirror, the pictures, the cornice, the chairs ; but we are deceived : being unconscious of the motions of the eye, and that each object is rapidly, but successively, presented to it. It is easy to show, that if the eye were steady, vision would be quickly lost : that all these objects, which are distinct and brilliant, are so from the motion of the eye : that they would disappear if it were otherwise. For example, let us fix the eye on one point, a thing difficult to do, owing to the very disposition to motion in the eye : but by repeated attempts we may at length acquire the power of fixing the eye to a point ; and when we have done so, we shall find, that the whole scene becomes more and more obscure, and finally vanishes. Let us fix the eye on the corner of the frame of the principal picture in the room. At first, every thing around it is distinct ; in a very little time, however, the impression becomes weaker, objects appear dim, and then the eye has an almost incontrollable desire to wander ; if this be resisted, the impressions of the figures in the picture first fade : for a time, we see the gilded frame : but this also becomes dim. When we have thus far ascertained the fact, we change the direction of the eye, but ever so little, and at once the whole scene is again perfect before us.

These phenomena are consequent upon the retina being subject to exhaustion. When a coloured ray of light impinges continuously on the same part of the retina, it becomess less sensible to it, but more sensible to a ray of the opposite colour. When the eye is fixed upon a point, the lights, shades, and colours of objects continuing to strike upon the same relative parts of the retina, the nerve is exhausted: but when the eye shifts, there is a new exercise of the nerve: the part of the retina that was opposed to the lights, is now opposed to the shades, and what was opposed to the different colours is now opposed to other colours, and the variation in the exciting cause produces a renewed sensation. From this it appears, how essential the incessant searching motion of the eye is to the continued exercise of the organ.

Before dismissing this subject, we may give another instance. If we are looking upon an extensive prospect, and have the eye caught by an object at a distance, or when, in expectation of a friend, we see a figure advancing on the distant road, and we endeavour to scrutinize the object, fixing the eye intently upon it, it disappears; in our disappointment we rub the eyes, cast them about, look again, and once more we see the object. The reason of this is very obvious: the retina is exhausted, but becomes recruited by looking on the other objects of different shades and colours. The sportsman on the moor or the hill side, feels this a hundred times when he marks down his covey, fixing his eye and travelling towards the spot.

Here we may interrupt our inquiry to observe how inconsistent these phenomena are with the favourite hypothesis—that light produces vision by exciting

vibration in the fibres of the nerve. By all the laws
of motion from which this hypothesis is borrowed,
we know that if a body be set in motion, it is easily
kept in motion ; and that if a cord vibrate, that vibration will be kept up by a motion in the same
time. It appears to me natural to suppose, that if
these fibres of the nerve (which, be it remembered,
are also imaginary) were moved like the cords of a
musical instrument, they would be most easily continued in motion by undulations in the same time :
that if the red ray oscillated or vibrated in a certain proportion of time, it would keep the fibres of the nerve
in action more easily, than a green ray, which vibrates in a different time. If the colour of a ray
depended upon the peculiar undulation or vibration,
it appears that before the green ray could produce a
motion corresponding with itself, it must encounter a
certain opposition, in interrupting the motion already
begun.*

* "Although any kind of impulse or motions regulated by any
" law may be transferred from molecule to molecule in an elastic
" medium, yet in the theory of light it is supposed that only such
" primary impulses, as recur according to regular periodical laws
" at equal intervals of time and repeated many times in succession, ·
" can affect our organs with the sensation of light. To put in motion
" the molecules of the nerves of our retina with sufficient efficacy,
" it is necessary that the almost infinitely minute impulse of the
" adjacent ethereal molecules should be often and regularly repeated,
" so as to multiply and concentrate their effect. Thus, as a great
" pendulum may be set in swing by a very minute force, often ap-
" plied at intervals exactly equal to its time of oscillation, or as one
" elastic body can be set in vibration, by the vibration of another at
" a distance propagated through the air, if in exact unison, even so
" we may conceive the gross fibres of the nerves of the retina to
" be thrown into motion by the continual repetition of the ethereal
" pulses ; and such only will be thus agitated, as from their size,
" shape or elasticity, are susceptible of vibrating in times exactly
" equal to those at which the impulses are repeated. Thus it is easy
" to conceive how the limits of visible colour may be established : for
" if there be no nervous fibres in unison with vibrations more or less
" frequent than certain limits, such vibrations, though they reach the
" retina, will produce no sensation. Thus, too, a single impulse, or
" an irregularly repeated one, produces no light. And thus also
" may the vibrations excited in the retina continue a sensible time af-

Reverting to the sensible spot in the retina, it does not appear that we are authorized in terming it a spot. The same law governs vision when we look to a fine point of a needle, or to an object in an extensive landscape. We look to the point of a pen, and we can rest the attention on the point upon the one side of the slit, to the exclusion of the other, just as we can select and intently survey a house or a tree. If the sensible spot were regularly defined, it must be very small : and were it, indeed, so defined, we should be sensible of it ; which we are not. The law, therefore, seems to be, at all times, that the nearer to the centre of the eye, the greater the sensibility to impression ; and this holds whether we are looking abroad in the country, or are microscopically intent upon objects of great minuteness.

When men deny the fine muscular adaptation of the eye to the sensation on the retina, how do they account for the obvious fact—that the eye-ball does move in such just degrees ? how is the one eye adjusted to the other with such marvellous precision? and how do the eyes move together in pursuit of an object, never failing to accompany it correctly, be it the flight of a bird, or the course of a tennis-ball, or even of a bomb-shell ? Is it not an irresistible conclusion—that if we so follow an object, adjusting the muscles of the eye so as to present the axis of vision successively to it, as it changes place, we must be sensible of these motions ? for how can we direct the muscles unless we be sensible to their action ? The question then comes, to be—whether being sensible to the condition of the muscles, and being capable of directing them with this extraordinary minuteness, this action of the

" ter the exciting cause has ceased, prolonging the sensation of light " (especially if a vivid one) for an instant in the eye in the manner " described." Sir W. Herschell, Art. Light. Enc. Met.

Now it does appear to me that this reasoning is inconsistent with the phenomena above noticed.

muscles does not enter into our computation of the place of an object? But is not this exactly the same question recurring as when we asked—whether we can direct the hand without knowing where the hand is? Must there not be a feeling or knowledge of the position of the hand, before we can give it direction to an object? And must we not have a conception of the relation of the muscles and of the position of the axis of the eye, before we can alter its direction to fix it upon a new object?

It surprises me to find ingenious men refusing their assent to the opinion, that the operation of the muscles of the eye is necessary to perfect vision, when the gradual acquisition of the power may be seen in observing the awakening sense in the infant. When a bright object is withdrawn from the infant's eye, there is a blank expression in the features; and an excitement when the object is again presented. For a time, the shifting of the object is not attended with the searching action of the eye: but, by and bye, the eye follows it and looks around for it, when it is lost. In this gradual acquisition of power in the eye, there is an exact parallel to the acquisition of motion in the hand; and in both instances, we seek to join the experience obtained by means of the muscular motion with the impression on the proper nerve of sense.

Some maintain that our idea of the position of an object is implanted in the mind and independent of experience. We must acknowledge the possibility of this, had it been so provided. We see the young of some creatures with their vision thus perfect at the moment of their birth. But in these animals, every corresponding faculty is, in the same manner, perfect from the beginning: the dropped foal, or the lamb, rises and follows its mother. We must no more compare the helpless human offspring with the young of these animals than with a fly, the existence of which is limited to an hour at noon,—which breaking from its confinement, knows its mate and deposits its eggs on the appropriate tree—the willow or the thorn, and dies. But this is foreign to our enquiry ; since it is obvious that the human eye has no such original power of vision bestowed upon it, and that it is acquired, as the exercise of the other senses, and the faculties of the mind itself are, by repeated efforts, or experience.

If it be admitted that the ideas which we receive through the eye come by experience, we must allow that the mind must be exercised in the act of comparison, before we can have a conception of any thing being exterior to the eye, or of an object being placed in a particular direction. Authors make the matter complex by conceiving a picture to be drawn at the bottom of the eye, and presenting to us the mind contemplating this inverted picture, and comparing the parts of it. But this leaves the subject without any explanation at all, and does not show how it is that the mind looks into this camera. The question will be, at least, more simple, if we consider the vision of a point ; and ask ourselves how we know the direction in which that point comes to the eye. Suppose it is a star in the heavens, or a beacon, seen by the mariner ; must he not, in order to ascertain the position of the star, find out some other object of comparison, some other star, which shall disclose to him the constellation to which the one that he is examining belongs : or to ascertain the position of the beacon, must he not look to his compass and card, and so trace the direction of the lighthouse in relation to them ? This is, in fact, the process that is followed in every thing which we see. A single point is directly in the axis of the eye, but we cannot judge of its position, without turning to some other point, and feeling sensible of the traversing of the eye-ball and the angle to which the eye is moved : or if we do not see another point to compare the first with, we must judge of its place by means of a comparison with the motion of the eye itself. We are sensible that the eye is directed to the right or to the left ; and we compare

17

the visible impression on the nerve with the motion, its direction, and its extent.

We find even mathematicians affirming that we judge of the direction of an object by the ray that falls upon the retina. But the ray which is here spoken of strikes a mere point of the retina : this point can have no direction ; the obliquity of the incidence of the ray can inform us of nothing : rays of all degrees of obliquity are converging to form that point. And do not the same mathematicians give us, in the first lessons of their science, as the definition of a line, that which is drawn through two points at the least ? Where are the two points here to indicate the direction of the line,—since the cornea, or the humours of the eye,* are not sensible to the passage of the ray ? Or is this an error which has crept in from inaccurate conceptions of the anatomy ? Has the idea that the direction of the ray can afford this knowledge, arisen from the notion that the ray passes through the thick and turbid matter of the retina ? I would ask for what reason is the "finder" attached to the great telescope ? is it not because the larger instrument from magnifying one object in a high degree, cannot be directed in the heavens, the observer seeing nothing but that one object ? Accordingly to remedy this, there is mounted on the greater telescope a smaller one, exactly parallel, of lesser power, but commanding a greater field : this finder, the astronomer directs to the constellation and moves from star to star, until that which he desires to examine is in the centre of the field : and by this means he adjusts the larger telescope to his object. Is this not a correct illustration of the operation of the eye ? is the eye not imperfectly exercised when it sees but one point—on the other hand, is it not in the full performance of its function when it moves from one object to the other,

---

* See a paper by Mr. Alexander Shaw, who has explained this subject very happily.—Journal of the Royal Institution, 1832.

judges of the degree and the direction of that motion,
and thus enables us, by comparison, to form our judgment ?

It has been stated by a most ingenious philosopher
of our own time, that the forms and relations of objects are known to us by the unassisted operation of
the eye-ball itself—by the transmission of the rays
through the humours of the eye, and by their effect
upon the retina ; and he has also affirmed that we
should know the position of objects even if the muscles
of the eye were paralytic. But I hope that it has
been understood, when I give so much importance to
the motions of the eye, that I do not neglect the
movements of the body, and, more especially, the
motions of the hand : that, in truth, the measure of
objects which we take through the eye, is in correspondence with the experience which we have had
through the motions of the whole frame, and that,
without such experience, we should have no knowledge of matter, or of position, or of distance, or of
form. Were the eye fixed in the head, or paralytic,
we should lose a great part of the exercise of the
organ, as well as all the appliances which are necessary for its protection : but we should still be capable
of comparing the visual impression with the experience of the body. As long as we know the right
hand from the left, or must raise our head to see what
is above us, or stoop to see a man's foot, there can be
no want of materials to form a comparison between
the impression on the nerve of sight and the experience of the body.

Against this view of the compound operation of
the eye, the matter is thus argued :—if a man receive
the impression of a luminous body upon his eye so
that the spectrum shall remain when the eye-lids
are shut, and if he be seated upon a stool that turns
round, and he be whirled round by the hand of a
friend, without his own effort, the motion of the spectrum will correspond with his own. No doubt it

will: because he is conscious of being turned round: a man cannot sit upon a stool that is turning without an effort to keep his place, without a consciousness of being turned round; and feeling, at the same time, that the impression is still before his eye, he will see the spectrum before him, and in that aspect to which he has been revolved.

Were I not conscious that I am right, I should feel it necessary to make an apology for differing from eminent men on this matter: but I conceive the explanation of this discrepancy to be, that we are very much influenced by the manner in which we approach to the examination of such a subject. A man lost in admiration of the properties of light, and of the effect of the humours of the eye as an optical instrument, may be blinded to those inferences, which to me seem so undeniable, accustomed as I have been to compare the properties of the eye with the living endowments of the frame. When instead of looking upon the eye as a mere camera or show box, with the picture inverted on the bottom, we determine the value of muscular activity; mark the sensation attending the balancing of the body; that fine property which we possess of adjusting the muscular frame to its various inclinations; how it is acquired in the child; how it is lost in the paralytic and drunkard; how motion and sensation are combined in the hand; how, in this way, the hand guides the finest instruments: when we consider how the eye and the hand correspond; how the motions of the eye, combining with the impression on the retina, become the means of measuring and estimating the place, form and distance of objects—the sign in the eye of what is known to the hand: finally, when, by attention to the motions of the eye, we are aware of their extreme minuteness, and how we are sensible to them in the finest degree—the conviction irresistibly follows, that without the power of directing the eye, (a motion holding relation to the action of the whole body) our finest organ of sense, which so largely contributes to the developement of the powers of the mind, would lie unexercised.

THE MOTION OF THE EYE CONSIDERED IN REGARD TO THE EFFECT OF SHADE AND COLOUR IN A PICTURE.

A QUESTION naturally arises whether it be possible, from this part of philosophy, to suggest some principles for the amateur and painter. The ideas and language of the amateur, when he attempts to establish rules for the disposition of colours or shades in a picture, are certainly very vague.

We have to remark, in the first place, that the colours of nature, and those of objects when represented in a painting, differ in most essential circumstances. Bodies of various colours, when placed together, have their colours reflected from the one to the other; and so they are sent to the eye. This is one mode in which the hues of nature are harmonized; but the colours upon the flat surface of the canvass cannot be thus reflected and mingled. The next difference results from the atmosphere, through which the rays from distant objects proceed to the eye and are softened; the canvass being near the eye, the effect which the atmosphere produces on colours amounts to nothing in the picture. The third mode in which colours are affected, is common to natural objects and to paintings, and is connected with the law of vision which we have been considering, and to which we must now revert.

When we make experiments by looking upon coloured spots, the effect on the sensibility of the retina is remarkable; and as this does not occur incidentally, but takes place, more or less, whenever we exercise the eye, it must have its influence when we look to works of art. The familiar fact which we have to carry with us into this enquiry, is, that if we throw a silver coin upon a dark table, and fix the eye upon the centre of it, when we remove the coin there is, for a moment, a white spot in its place, which presently becomes deep black. If we put a red wafer upon a sheet of paper, and look upon it, and continue to keep the eye fixed on the same point, upon removing the wafer, the spot where it lay on the white paper will appear green. If we look upon a green wafer in the same manner and remove it, the spot will be red; if upon blue or indigo, the paper will appear yellow. These phenomena are to be explained by considering that the nerve is exhausted by the continuance of the impression, and becomes more apt to receive sensation from an opposite colour. All the colours of the prism come into the eye from the surface of the paper when the wafer has been removed; but if the nerve has been exhausted by the incidence of the red rays upon it, it will be insensible to these red rays when they are thus reflected from the paper; the effect of the rays of an opposite kind will be increased, and consequently the spot will be no longer white, but of the prevailing green colour.

Let us see how the loss of sensibility produces an effect in engraving, where there is no colour, and only light and shade.

Is it possible that a high tower, in a cloudless sky, can be less illuminated at the top than at the bottom? Yet if we turn to a book of engravings, where an old steeple or tower is represented standing up against the clear sky, we shall find that all the higher part is dark, and that the effect is picturesque and pleasing. Now this is perfectly correct, for although the highest part of the tower be in the brightest illumination, it is not seen so—it never appears so to the eye. The reason is, that when we look to the steeple, a great part of the retina is opposed to the light of the sky; and on shifting the eye to look at the particular parts of the steeple, the reflected light from that object falls upon the retina, where it is exhausted by the direct light of the sky. If we look to the top of the tower, and then drop the eye to some of the lower architectural ornaments, the effect infallibly is that the upper half of the tower is dark. For example, if

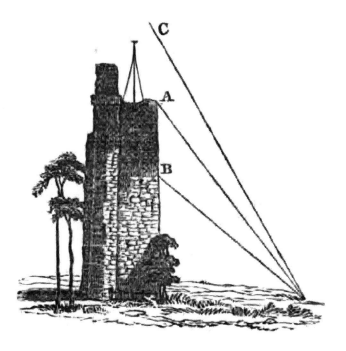

looking to the point A we drop the eye to B: the tower from A to B is seen by that part of the retina which was opposed to the clear sky from A to C; and it is dark not by contrast, as it would be thought-lessly said, but by the nerve being somewhat exhaust-ed of its sensibility. This, then, is the first effect we shall remark as arising from the searching motion of the eye.

The refreshing colours of the natural landscape are at no time so pleasing as when reading on a journey, we turn the eye from the book to the fields and woods; the shadows are then deeper—the greens more sooth-ing, and the whole colours are softened. Reynolds observed to Sir George Beaumont that the pictures of Rubens appeared different to him, and less brilliant, on his second visit to the continent; and the reason of the difference he discovered to be that, on the first visit, he had taken notes, and on the second he did not. The alleged reason is quite equal to the effect; but I cannot help imagining that there is some incorrectness in the use of the term brilliant, unless warmth and depth of colouring is meant, for when the eye turns from the white paper to the painting, the reds and yellows must necessarily be deeper. If we look out from the window, and then turn towards a picture, the whole effect is gone—the reflected rays from the picture are too feeble to produce their impression; and if we look upon a sheet of paper, and then upon a picture, the tone will be deeper, and the warm tints stronger, but the lights and shades less distinct. If we place an oil painting without the frame, upon a large sheet of paper, or against a white plastered wall, it is offensively yellow. Here the eye alternately, though insensibly, moving from the white paper or wall to the painting, which is of a deep tone, the browns and yellows are unnaturally strong. We see the necessity or the effect of the gilt frame for such a picture: it does not merely cut off surrounding objects, but it prepares the eye for the colours of the painting—it allows, if I may so express it, the painter to use his art more boldly, and to exaggerate the colours of nature.

Painters proceed by experiment. If they are painting a portrait, they may represent the features by contrasts of lights and shadows with very little colour; but such a portrait is never popular. If they are to represent the features without much contrast of light and shade, they must raise the features by contrasts of colours, and the carnations are necessarily exaggerated; but all this is softened down by throwing a piece of drapery into the picture, the colours of which so prepare the eye that, now looking on the features, that will appear natural, which, but for this art, would have represented an inflamed countenance. The common resource of the painter is to throw in a crimson curtain, or to introduce some flower or piece of dress, that shall lead the eye, by a succession of tints, or, more accurately speaking, shall prepare the eye to receive the otherwise exaggerated colours of the portrait. The eye cast on the red curtain, and then falling on the countenance, sees it as if coloured only with the modesty of nature.

Those who hang pictures, do not place an historical picture, painted after the manner of the Bolognese school with distinct and abrupt coloured draperies, by the side of a landscape ; for the colours of a landscape, to be at all consonant with nature, are weak and reduced to a low tone, by representing that effect, which we observed, of the intervention of the atmosphere. The colours, therefore, would be destroyed by too powerful a contrast. There is a difficulty of deciding what should be the colour of the walls of a gallery, because the pictures are, for the most part, painted on different principles ; but generally speaking, the dark subdued red or morone colour brings out the colours of paintings ; in other words, if we look on a wall of this colour, and then turn to the picture, the prevailing green and yellow tints will appear brighter.

The word " contrast" is used without a definition, or without the actual comprehension of what it means. Now the effect of colours, on being placed together, is produced through the *motion* of the eye, combined with this law of the sensibility of the retina, which we have been adverting to. When we imagine that we are comparing colours, we are really experiencing the effect of the nerve being exhausted, by dwelling on one colour, and made more susceptible of the opposite colour. In coloured drapery, for example, there is such a mixture of all colours reflected from it, although one prevails, that the impression may be greatly modified by what the eye has previously experienced. If the colouring of the flesh be, as the painter terms it, "too warm," it may be made "cold" by rendering the eye insensible to the red and yellow rays, and more than usually susceptible of the blue and purple rays. Every coloured ray from the flesh is transmitted to the eye ; but if the eye has moved to it from a yellow or crimson drapery, then the rays of that kind will be, for the moment, lost to the vision, and the colour of the flesh will appear less warm, in consequence of the prevalence of the opposite rays of colour.

It ought to be unsatisfactory to the philosophical student to make use of a term without knowing its full meaning. There has been a great deal said about contrast and harmony in painting, as resulting from certain colours placed together—the idea being that we see these colours at the same time—whereas, the effect, of which we are all sensible, results from alternately looking at the one and at the other. The subject might be pleasantly pursued, but I mean only to vindicate the importance of the motions of the eye to our enjoyment, whether of the colours of art or of nature. There is another subject of some interest, namely, the effect produced upon the retina when the eye is intently fixed upon an object, and is not permitted to wander from point to point. This touches the chiaroscuro of painting ; which is not merely the managing of the lights and-shadows, but the preserving of the parts of a scene subordinate to the principal object. There is something unpleasant and imperfect, even to the least experienced eye, in a picture in which every thing is made out—the drapery of every figure, the carving or ornament of every object minutely represented ; for these things were never so seen in nature. The true picture, on the other hand, is effective, and felt to be natural, when the eye is at once led to dwell on that principal group, or principal figure, with which it is the artist's intention to occupy the imagination. By fine mastery of his art, and by insensible degrees, the painter keeps down the parts which are removed from the centre; and thus he represents the scene as when we look intently upon an object—seeing that which is near the axis of the eye distinctly—the other objects, as it were, retreating or rising out less and less distinctly, in proportion as they recede from the centre. In the one instance, the artist paints a panorama, where we turn round and have presented before the eye the several divisions of the circle, in each of which the objects are equally distinct; in the other, he paints a picture representing things, not as when the eye wanders from the one part to the other, but where it is fixed with higher interest upon some central object, while the others fall off subordinately.

Looking to our main argument, the proofs of beneficence in the capacities of the living frame, we revert naturally to the pleasures received through this double property of the eye—motion and sensibility; and whilst we perceive that the varieties of light and shade are necessary to vision, we find that the coloured rays are also, by variety, suited to the higher exercise of this sense. They do not all equally illuminate objects, nor are they all equally agreeable to the eye. The yellow, pale green, or Isabella colours, illuminate in the highest degree, and are the most agreeable to the sense; and we cannot but observe, on looking out on the face of nature, that they are the prevailing colours.* The red ray illuminates the least, but it irritates the most; and it is this variety in the influence of these rays upon the nerve that continues its exercise, and adds so much to our enjoyment. We have pleasure from the succession and contrast of colours, independently of that higher gratification which the mind enjoys through the influence of association.

---

* The astronomer selects a glass for his telescope, which refracts the pale yellow light in the greatest proportion, because it illuminates in the highest degree and irritates the least.

ADDITIONAL ILLUSTRATIONS TO THE CONCLUDING CHAPTER.

I HAVE sometimes thought it possible, that a greatly extended survey of nature may humble too much our conceptions of ourselves; and that this requires to be corrected by the study of things more minute, and in which we are more directly concerned : by dwelling on the perfection of the frame of the animal body and the marvellous endowments of the living properties. When we have formed some estimate of the immensity of the heavenly bodies, we are struck with admiration in following the successive advancement made in the science :—an improvement in the curves of the glasses of the telescope, a new mode of polishing the reflecting surfaces, a change in the chemical composition of the glasses, or a more perfect adjustment of their dispersive powers—is followed by the discovery of circle beyond circle of worlds interminably.

We fan the imagination and labour to comprehend the immensity of the creation, and fall back with the impression of the littleness of all that belongs to us: our lives seem but a point of time, compared with the astronomical and geological periods, and we ourselves as atoms, driven about, amidst unceasing changes of the material world.

But it has been shown, that whether we take the animal body as a single machine, or embrace in the survey the successive creation of animals, conforming always to the improving condition of the earth, there is nothing like chance or irregularity in the composition of the system. In proportion indeed as we comprehend the principles of mechanics, or of hydraulics, as applicable to the animal machinery, we shall be satisfied of the perfection of the design: and if any thing appear disjointed or thrown in by chance, let the student mark that for contemplation and experiment, and most certainly when it comes to be understood, other parts will receive the illumination, and the whole design stand more fully disclosed.

The extension of knowledge has not necessarily the effect of raising the mind to more consolatory contemplations. We may quote the ancient philosopher in contrast with the modern. The former having nothing in his mind to draw him from observing the just relations of human beings to the world; but on the contrary, seeing every thing suited to man or subordinate, thinks of him "as a little God harboured in a humane body." But when by science, and the aid of instruments, or "the ingenuity of the hand," vision is extended to things too remote perhaps, or too minute, to fall within our natural sphere; when instead of the extended plane, and visible horizon of the stable earth, it is thought of as a ball rolling through space, amidst myriads besides, greater than it: the expression is excusable that—" the earth with man upon it does not seem much other than an ant-hill, where some ants carry corn, and some carry their young, and some go empty, and all to and fro, a little heap of dust."

We may consider man, before the lights of modern philosophy had their influence on his thoughts, as in a state more natural; in as much as he yielded unresistingly to those sentiments which directly flow from the objects and phenomena around him. But when that period of society arrived, in which man made natural phenomena the subjects of experiment or of philosophical enquiry, then was there some danger of a change of opinion, not always beneficial to his state of mind. This danger does not touch the philosopher so much as the scholar. He who has strength of mind and ingenuity enough to make investigations into

18

nature, will not be satisfied with the discovery of secondary causes—his mind will be enlarged, and the subjects of his thoughts and aspirations become more elevated.   But it is otherwise with those not themselves habituated to investigation, and who learn at second-hand, the result of those enquiries.   If such a one sees the fire of heaven brought down into a phial, and the materials compounded, to produce an explosion louder than the thunder, and ten times more destructive, the storm will no longer speak a language to him.   Those influences which are natural and just, and beneficently provided, and have served to develope the sentiments of millions before him, are dismissed as things vulgar and to be despised.—Yet with all the pride of newly acquired knowledge, his conceptions embarrass, if they do not mislead him ; in short, he has not had that intellectual discipline, which should precede and accompany the acquisition of knowledge.

But a man, possessed of genius of the highest order, may lose the just estimate of himself, from another cause.   The sublime nature of his studies may consign him to depressing thoughts.   He may forget the very attributes of his mind, which have privileged these high contemplations, and the ingenuity of the hand, which has so extended the sphere of his observation.

The remedy, to such a mind, is in the studies which we are enforcing.   The heavenly bodies, in their motions through space, are held in their orbits by the continuence of a power, not more wonderful nor more deserving of admiration, than that, by which a globule of blood is suspended in the mass of fluids :—or by which, in due season, it is attracted and resolved : than that, by which a molecule entering into the composition of the body, is driven through a circle of revolutions, and made to undergo different states of aggregation ; becoming sometime, a part of a fluid, sometime, an ingredient of a solid :—and finally cast out again, from the influence of the living forces.

Our argument in the early part of the volume, has shown man, by the power of the hand (as the ready instrument of the mind) accommodated to every condition through which his destinies promise to be accomplished. We first see the hand ministering to his necessities, and sustaining the life of the individual :—a second stage of his progress, we see it adapted to the wants of society, when man becomes a labourer and an artificer. In a state still more advanced, science is brought in aid of mechanical ingenuity. The elements which seemed adverse to the progress of society, become the means conducing to it. The seas which at first set limits to nations, and grouped mankind into families, are now the means by which they are associated. Philosophical chemistry has subjected the elements to man's use ; and all tend to the final accomplishment of the great objects to which every thing, from the beginning, has pointed : the multiplication and distribution of mankind, and the enlargement of the sources of his comfort and enjoyment—the relief from too incessant toil, and the consequent improvement of the higher faculties of his nature. Instinct has directed animals, until they are spread to the utmost verge of their destined places of abode. Man too is borne onwards ; and although, on consulting his reason, much is dark and doubtful, yet does his genius operate to fulfil the same design, enlarging the sphere of life and enjoyment.

Whilst we have before us the course of human advancement, as in a map, we are recalled to a narrower, and yet a more important consideration : for what to us avail all these proofs of divine power—of harmony in nature—of design—the predestined accommodation of the earth, and the creation of man's frame and faculties, if we are stopped here ? If we perceive no more direct relation between the individual and the Creator ? But we are not so precluded from advancement : on the contrary, reasons accumulate at every step, for a higher estimate of the living soul, and give

us assurance that its condition is the final object and
end of all this machinery, and of these successive
revolutions.

To this, must be referred the weakness of the frame,
and its liability to injury, the helplessness of infancy,
the infirmities of age, the pains, diseases, distresses,
and afflictions of life—for by such means is man to
be disciplined—his faculties and virtues unfolded, and
his affections drawn to a spiritual Protector.

THE

CLASSIFICATION OF ANIMALS,

IN EXPLANATION OF THE TERMS INCIDENTALLY USED IN THE VOLUME.

———

THE ANIMAL KINGDOM is arranged in four Divisions:

Division I. *Vertebral Animals :* so called from their possessing a vertebral column or spine.

Division II. *Molluscous Animals :* such as shell-fish, which are of a soft structure, and without a skeleton. *Etym.* mollis, soft.

Division III. *Articulated Animals :* like the worm or insect : they are without a skeleton, but their skins or coverings are divided and jointed. *Etym.* Articulus, dim. a joint.

Division IV. *Zoophytes :* animals believed to be composed very nearly of a homogeneous pulp, which is moveable and sensible, and resembles the form of a plant. *Etym.* ζωον, zoon, a living creature ; φυτόν, phyton, a plant.

DIVISION I.

The division of vertebral animals is composed of four Classes : viz., 1. Mammalia, animals which suckle their young. *Etym.* mamma, a teat. 2. Aves. *Etym.* avis, a bird. 3. Reptilia, animals that crawl. *Etym.* from a part of the word repo, to creep. 4. Pisces. *Etym.* piscis, a fish.

The first Class Mammalia, is divided into Orders, which are subdivided into Genera, and these are further divided into Species.

We present the principal Orders with familiar examples.

Bimana, man. *Etym.* bis, double ; manus, hand.

18*

Quadrumana. *Etym.* quatuor, four; manus, hand. Monkeys, makis or lemurs (*Etym.* lemures, ghosts.) The loris tardigradus (tardus, slow; gradior, to walk) is a species of lemur.

Cheiroptera. *Etym.* χειρ, *cheir*, the hand; πτερον, pteron, a wing. The Bats.

Insectivora. *Etym.* insecta, insects; voro, to eat. Hedge-hog; shrew; mole.

Plantigrade. *Etym.* planta, the sole of the foot; gradior, to walk. Bear; racoon.

Digitigrade. *Etym.* digitus, the toe, or finger; gradior, to walk. Lion; wolf; dog; weasel.

Amphibia. *Etym.* αμφι, *amphi*, both; βιος, *bios*, life. Walrus; seal.

Marsupialia. *Etym.* marsupium, a pouch. Kangaroo; opossum.

Rodentia. *Etym.* rodo, to gnaw. Squirrel; beaver; rat; hare.

Edentata. *Etym.* edentulus, toothless: animals without the front teeth. Ai; unau; armadillo; ant-eater; tamandua; megatherium (μεγα, *mega*, great; θηριον, *therion*, a wild beast); megalonyx (μεγας, *megas*, great; ονυξ, *onyx*, a claw); ornithorhynchus (ορνιθος; *ornithos*, of a bird; ρυγχος, *rhynchos*, a beak.)

Pachydermata. *Etym.* παχυς, *pachys*, thick; δερμα, *derma*, skin. Rhinoceros, elephant; mammoth: mastodon (μαστος, *mastos*, a nipple; οδων, *odon*, a tooth); tapir; horse; couagga.

Ruminantia. *Etym.* ruminatio, chewing the cud. Camel; giraffe; deer; goat; cow; sheep.

Cetacea. *Etym.* cetus, a whale. Dolphin; whale; dugong.

SECOND CLASS. *Aves, or Birds.*

Accipitres. *Etym.* accipiter, a hawk. Vulture; eagle; owl.

Passeres. *Etym.* passer, a sparrow. Lark; thrush; swallow; crow; wren.

Scansores. *Etym.* scando, to climb. Parrot; wood-pecker; toucan.

Gallinæ. *Etym.* gallina, a hen. Peacock; pheasant; pigeon.

Grallæ. *Etym.* grallæ, stilts. Ostrich; stork; ibis; flamingo.

Palmipedes. *Etym.* palma, the palm of the hand; pes, foot. Swan; pelican; gull.

THIRD CLASS. *Reptiles.*

Chelonia. *Etym.* χελυς, *chelys*, a tortoise. Tortoise; turtle.

Sauria. *Etym.* σαυρα, *saura*, a lizard. Crocodile; alligator, chameleon; dragon; pterdoctyle (πτερον, *pteron*, a wing: δακτυλος, *dacty-*

lus, a finger) ; ichthyosaurus (*ιχθυς, ichthys*, a fish ; *σαυρα, saura*, a lizard) ; plesiosaurus (*πλεσιον, plesion*, near to ; *σαυρα, saura*, a reptile) ; megalasaurus (*μεγαλη, megale*, great ; *σαυρα, saura*, a reptile) ; iguanadon.

Ophidia. *Etym. οφις, ophis*, a serpent. Boa ; viper.

Batrachia. *Etym. βατραχος, batrachos*, a frog. Frog ; salamander ; proteus.

FOURTH CLASS. *Fishes.*

Chondropterygii. *Etym. χονδρος, chondros*, gristle ; *πτερυξ, pterys*, the ray of a fin. Ray ; sturgeon ; shark ; lamprey ; ammocete (*αμμος, ammos*, sand ; *κητος, cetos*, a fish.)

Plectognathi. *Etym. πλεκω, pleco*, to join ; *γναθος, gnathos*, the jaw. Sun-fish ; trunk-fish.

Lophobranchi. *Etym. λοφος, lophos*, a loop ; *βραγχια, branchia*, the gills. Pipe-fish ; pegasus.

Melacopterygii. *Etym. μαλακος, malakos*, soft ; *πτερυξ, pterys*, the ray of a fin. Salmon ; trout ; cod ; herring ; remora.

Acanthopterygii. *Etym. ακανθα, acantha*, a thorn ; *πτερυξ, pterys*, the ray of a fin. Perch ; sword-fish ; mackarel ; lophius piscatorius (*λοφια, lophia*, a pennant ; piscator, a fisher) ; chætodon rostratus (*χαιτε, chæte*, hair ; *οδων, odon*, a tooth ; rostratus, beaked) ; zeus ciliaris (cilium, an eye-lash.)

DIVISION II.

MOLLUSCOUS ANIMALS.

1st Class. Cephalopoda. *Etym. κεφαλε, cephale*, the head ; *ποδα, poda*, the feet. Animals which have their organs of motion arranged round their head.

This Class includes Sepia, or Cuttle-fish. Argonauts (*Αργω*, the ship Argo, *ναυτης, nautes*, a sailor). Nautilus, (*ναυτης, nautes*, a sailor.) Ammonite, an extinct Cephalopode which inhabited a shell resembling that of the Nautilus ; coiled like the horns of a ram or of the statues of Jupiter Ammon ; whence the name. Belemnites : also extinct : the shell is long, straight, and conical (*βελεμνον, belemnon*, a dart). Nummulites : likewise extinct. Whole chains of rocks are formed of its shells. The pyramids of Egypt are built of these rocks, (nummus, a coin).

2nd Class. Pteropoda. *Etym. πτερον, pteron*, a wing ; *ποδα, poda*, feet ; having fins or processes resembling wings on each side of the mouth.

The Clio Borealis, which abounds in the North Seas, and is the principal food of the whale.

3rd Class. Gasteropoda. *Etym.* γαστηρ, *gaster*, the stomach; ποδα, *poda*, the feet. Animals which move by means of a fleshy apparatus placed under the belly.

The snail; slug; limpet.

4th Class. Acephala. *Etym.* α, α, without; κεφαλη, *cephale*, the head. Molluscous animals without a head.

The oyster; muscle.

5th Class. Brachiopoda. *Etym.* βραχιον, *brachion*, the arm; ποδα, *poda*, the feet. Animals which move by means of processes like arms.

Lingula; terebratula.

6th Class. Cirrhopoda. *Etym.* cirrus, a lock or tuft of hair; ποδα, *poda*, the feet.

Balanus; barnacle · anatifera, (anas, a duck, fero, to bring forth.)

DIVISION III.

ARTICULATA.

1st Class. Annelides, or Vermes. *Etym. Annellus*, a little ring; *vermis*, a worm.

Leech; sea-mouse; earth-worm; sand-worm; tubicolæ, (tubus, a tube, colo, to inhabit); worms which cover themselves by means of a slimy secretion that exudes from their surfaces, with a case of small shells and pebbles, like the caddis-worm, or with sand and mud.

2nd Class. Crustacea. Animals which have a shelly crust, covering their bodies.

The crabs; shrimps; lobsters.

3rd Class. Arachnida. *Etym.* αραχνης, *arachnes*, a spider.

Spiders; aranea scenica, or saltica; the leaping spider; the scorpion spider; the mite.

4th Class. Insecta. They are divided into insects which are without wings and those which have them: and these are further subdivided according to the peculiarities of the wings.

Aptera (α, α, without; πτερον, *pteron*, a wing.) Centipede (having a hundred feet); louse; flea.

Coleoptera (κολεος, *coleos*, a sheath or scabbard, πτερον, a wing), insects which have their wings protected by a cover, as the beetle, corn-weevil. *Orthoptera* (ορθος, *orthos*, straight, πτερον), as the locust, grass-hopper. *Hemiptera* (ἡμισυ, *hemisu*, half, πτερον), insects which have one half of their wings thick and coriaceous, and the other membranous ; such as a bug, tick, fire-fly. *Neuroptera* (νευρον, *neuron*, a nerve, πτερον), dragon-fly ; ant-lion ; ephemera. *Hymenoptera* (ὑμεν, *hymen*, a membrane, πτερον), the bee ; wasp ; ant. *Lepidoptera* (λεπις, *lepis*, a scale, πτερον), moth ; butter-fly. *Rhipiptera* (ῥιπις, *ripis*, a fan, πτερον), xenos ; stylops. *Diptera* (δις, *dis* double, πτερον), house-fly ; gnat.

DIVISION IV.

ZOOPHYTES.

Echinodermata (*Etym.* εχινος, *echinos*, a hedgehog ; δερμα, *derma*, the skin), the star-fish ; sea urchin. *Entoza* (εντος, *entos*, within ; ζαω *zao*, to live), tænia hydatia. *Acalephæ* (ακαληφη, *acalephe*, a nettle), medusa ; polypi (containing much sap ; sea-anemone ; hydra ; tubipora (inhabiting tubes) ; sertularia ; cellularia ; flustra ; coralline ; sponge. *Infusoria* (found in infusions or stagnant water), monas ; vibrio ; proteus.

THE END.

BRIDGEWATER TREATISES.

This series of Treatises is published under the following circumstances:—

The Right Honorable and Rev. FRANCIS HENRY, Earl of Bridgewater, died in the month of February, 1825; he directed certain trustees therein named, to invest in the public funds, the sum of eight thousand pounds sterling; this sum, with the accruing dividends thereon, to be held at the disposal of the President, for the time being, of the Royal Society of London, to be paid to the person or persons nominated by him. The Testator farther directed, that the person or persons selected by the said President, should be appointed to write, print and publish one thousand copies of a work, on the Power, Wisdom, and Goodness of God, as manifested in the Creation; illustrating such work, by all reasonable arguments, as, for instance, the variety and formation of God's creatures in the Animal, Vegetable, and Mineral Kingdoms; the effect of digestion, and, thereby, of conversion; the construction of the hand of man, and an infinite variety of other arguments; as also by discoveries, ancient and modern, in arts, sciences, and the whole extent of literature.

He desired, moreover, that the profits arising from the sale of the works so published, should be paid to the authors of the works.

The late President of the Royal Society, DAVIES GILBERT, Esq. requested the assistance of his Grace, the Archbishop of Canterbury, and of the Bishop of London, in determining upon the best mode of carrying into effect, the intentions of the Testator. Acting with their advice, and with the concurrence of a nobleman immediately connected with the deceased, Mr. Davies Gilbert appointed the following eight gentlemen to write separate Treatises in the different branches of the subjects here stated:—

I. The Adaptation of External Nature to the Moral and Intellectual Constitution of Man, by the Rev. THOMAS CHALMERS, D. D., Professor of Divinity in the University of Edinburgh.

II. The adaptation of External Nature to the Physical Condition of Man, by JOHN KIDD, M. D., F. R. S., Regius Professor of Medicine in the University of Oxford.

III. Astronomy and General Physics, considered with reference to Natural Theology, by the Rev. Wm. Whewell, M. A., F. R. S., Fellow of Trinity College, Cambridge.

IV. The hand: its mechanism and vital endowments as evincing design, by Sir Charles Bell, K. H., F. R. S.

V. Animal and Vegetable Physiology, by Peter Mark Roget, M. D., Fellow of and Secretary to the Royal Society.

VI. Geology and Mineralogy, by the Rev. Wm. Buckland, D. D., F. R. S., Canon of Christ Church, and Professor of Geology in the University of Oxford.

VII. The History, Habits, and Instincts of Animals, by the Rev. Wm. Kirby, M. A., F. R. S.

BRIDGEWATER TREATISES.

VIII. Chemistry, Meteorology, and the Function of Digestion, by Wm. Prout, M. D., F. R. S.

THE FOLLOWING ARE PUBLISHED.

ASTRONOMY AND GENERAL PHYSICS, considered with reference to Natural Theology. By the Rev. WILLIAM WHEWELL, M. A., Fellow and Tutor of Trinity College, Cambridge; being Part III. of the Bridgewater Treatises on the Power, Wisdom, and Goodness of God, as manifested in the Creation. In one vol. 12mo.

" It is a work of profound investigation, deep research, distinguished alike for the calm Christian spirit which breathes throughout, and the sound, irresistible argumentation which is stamped on every page."—*Daily Intelligencer.*

" Let works like that before us be widely disseminated, and the bold, active, and ingenious enemies of religion be met by those, equally sagacious, alert and resolute, and the most timid of the many who depend upon the few, need not fear the host that comes with subtle steps to 'steal their faith away.' "—*N. Y. American.*

" That the devoted spirit of the work is most exemplary, that we have here and there found, or fancied, room for cavil, only peradventure because we have been unable to follow the author through the prodigious range of his philosophical survey—and in a word, that the work before us would have made the reputation of any other man, and may well maintain even that of Professor Whewell."—*Metropolitan.*

" He has succeeded admirably in laying a broad foundation, in the light of nature, for the reception of the more glorious truths of revelation ; and has produced a work well calculated to dissipate the delusions of scepticism and infidelity, and to confirm the believer in his faith."—*Charleston Courier.*

" The known talents, and high reputation of the author, gave an earnest of excellence, and nobly has Mr. Whewell redeemed the pledge.—In conclusion, we have no hesitation in saying, that the present is one of the best works of its kind, and admirably adapted to the end proposed ; as such, we cordially recommend it to our readers."—*London Lit. Gazette.*

" It is a work of high character."—*Boston Recorder.*

A TREATISE ON THE ADAPTATION OF EXTERNAL NATURE TO THE PHYSICAL CONDITION OF MAN, principally with reference to the supply of his wants, and the exercise of his intellectual faculties. By JOHN KIDD, M. D., F. R. S., Regius Professor of Medicine in the University of Oxford; being Part II. of the Bridgewater Treatises on the Power, Wisdom, and Goodness of God, as manifested in the Creation. In one vol. 12mo.

" It is ably written, and replete both with interest and instruction. The diffusion of such works cannot fail to be attended with the happiest effects in justifying 'the ways of God to man,' and illustrating the wisdom and goodness of the Creator by arguments which appeal irresistably both to the reason and the feelings. Few can understand abstract reasoning, and still fewer relish it, or will listen to it : but in this work the purest morality and the kindliest feelings are inculcated through the medium of agreeable and useful information."—*Balt. Gaz.*

" It should be in the hands of every individual who feels disposed to ' vindicate the ways of God to man.' "—*N. Y. Com. Adv.*

BRIDGEWATER TREATISES.

"No one will read this book without profit; it is certainly one of the most interesting volumes we have ever read."—*Philadelphia Gazette.*

"Dr. Kidd has fulfilled his task, and may claim the gratitude of those who delight to contemplate the wisdom of Providence in the works of nature, and to discover the adaptation of the vegetable to the animal world, and the subserviency of the whole to the high destinies of man."—*U. S. Gazette.*

"The subject has been ably treated by a learned professor, and though it is not the most captivating topic in the world, has certainly served to display the ability of a sound thinker, who might rise, on other themes, to eloquence."—*Sat. Evening Post.*

"We congratulate Professor Kidd on the production of his work, and repeat the commendation, to which, as a popular treatise, it is indisputably entitled."—*Christian Remembrancer.*

ON THE ADAPTATION OF EXTERNAL NATURE TO THE MORAL AND INTELLECTUAL CONSTITUTION OF MAN. By the Rev. THOMAS CHALMERS, D. D.; being Part I. of the Bridgewater Treatises on the Power, Wisdom, and Goodness of God, as manifested in the Creation. In one vol. 12mo.

"The volumes before us are every way worthy of their subject. It would seem almost supererogetary to pass any judgment on the style of a writer so celebrated as Dr. Chalmers. He is well known as a logician not to be baffled by any difficulties; as one who boldly grapples with his theme, and brings every energy of his clear and nervous intellect into the field. No sophistry escapes his eagle visions—no argument that could either enforce or illustrate his subject is left untouched. Our literature owes a deep debt of gratitude to the author of these admirable volumes."—*Lit. Gazette.*

THE HAND: ITS MECHANISM AND VITAL ENDOWMENTS, AS EVINCING DESIGN. By Sir CHARLES BELL, K. G. H.; being Part IV. of the Bridgewater Treatises on the Power, Wisdom, and Goodness of God, as manifested in the Creation. In one vol. 12mo.

SOCIETY AND MANNERS
IN GREAT BRITAIN AND IRELAND.

By the Rev. C. S. STEWART, U. S. Navy, Author of A Voyage to the South Seas, &c. In 2 vols. 12mo. In the press.

MEN AND MANNERS IN AMERICA.

By Major HAMILTON, Author of Cyril Thornton, Annals of Peninsular Campaigns, &c. In 1 vol. 8vo.

MEDICINE.

THE PRACTICE OF PHYSIC. By W. P. DEWEES, M. D., Adjunct Professor of Midwifery, in the University of Pennsylvania. New edition, greatly enlarged, complete in one vol. 8vo.

"We have no hesitation in recommending it as decidedly one of the best systems of medicine extant. The tenor of the work in general reflects the highest honor on Dr. Dewees's talents, industry, and capacity for the execution of the arduous task which he had undertaken. It is one of the most able and satisfactory works which modern times have produced, and will be a standard authority."—*London Med. and Surg. Journal, Aug.* 1830.

DEWEES ON THE DISEASES OF CHILDREN. 5th ed. In 8vo.

The objects of this work are, 1st, to teach those who have the charge of children, either as parent or guardian, the most approved methods of securing and improving their physical powers. This is attempted by pointing out the duties which the parent or the guardian owes for this purpose, to this interesting, but helpless class of beings, and the manner by which their duties shall be fulfilled. And 2d, to render available a long experience to these objects of our affection when they become diseased. In attempting this, the author has avoided as much as possible, "technicality;" and has given, if he does not flatter himself too much, to each disease of which he treats, its appropriate and designating characters, with a fidelity that will prevent any two being confounded together, with the best mode of treating them, that either his own experience or that of others has suggested.

DEWEES ON THE DISEASES OF FEMALES. 4th edition, with Additions. In 8vo.

A COMPENDIOUS SYSTEM OF MIDWIFERY; chiefly designed to facilitate the Inquiries of those who may be pursuing this Branch of Study. By W. P. DEWEES, M. D. In 8vo. with 13 Plates. Sixth edition, corrected and enlarged.

THE ELEMENTS OF THERAPEUTICS AND MATERIA MEDICA. By N. CHAPMAN, M. D. 2 vols. 8vo. 5th edition, corrected and revised.

MANUAL OF PATHOLOGY: containing the Symptoms, Diagnosis, and Morbid Character of Diseases, &c. By L. MARTINET. Translated, with Notes and Additions, by JONES QUAIN. Second American Edition, 12mo.

"We strongly recommend M. Martinet's Manual to the profession, and especially to students; if the latter wish to study diseases to advantage, they should always have it at hand, both when at the bedside of the patient, and when making post mortem examinations."—*American Journal of the Medical Sciences, No. I.*

CLINICAL ILLUSTRATIONS OF FEVER, comprising a Report of the Cases treated at the London Fever Hospital in 1828-29, by Alexander Tweedie, M. D., Member of the Royal College of Physicians of London, &c. 1 vol. 8vo.

"In short, the present work, concise, unostentatious as it is, would have led us to think that Dr. Tweedie was a man of clear judgment, unfettered by attachment to any fashionable hypothesis, that he was an energetic but judicious practitioner, and that, if he did not dazzle his readers with the brilliancy of theoretical speculations he would command their assent to the solidity of his didactic precepts."—*Med. Chir. Journal.*

MEDICINE.

THE ANATOMY, PHYSIOLOGY, AND DISEASES OF THE TEETH. By THOMAS BELL, F. R. S., F. L. S. &c. In 1 vol. 8vo. With Plates.

"Mr. Bell has evidently endeavored to construct a work of reference for the practitioner, and a text-book for the student, containing a 'plain and practical digest of the information at present possessed on the subject, and results of the author's own investigations and experience.'" * * * "We must now take leave of Mr. Bell, whose work we have no doubt will become a class-book on the important subject of dental surgery."—*Medico-Chirurgical Review.*

"We have no hesitation in pronouncing it to be the best treatise in the English language."—*North American Medical and Surgical Journal, No.* 19.

AMERICAN DISPENSATORY. Ninth Edition, improved and greatly enlarged. By JOHN REDMAN COXE, M. D. Professor of Materia Medica and Pharmacy in the University of Pennsylvania. In 1 vol. 8vo.

⁎ This new edition has been arranged with special reference to the recent Pharmacopœias, published in Philadelphia and New-York.

ELLIS' MEDICAL FORMULARY. The Medical Formulary, being a collection of prescriptions derived from the writings and practice of many of the most eminent Physicians in America and Europe. By BENJAMIN ELLIS, M. D. 3d. edition. With Additions.

"We would especially recommend it to our brethren in distant parts of the country, whose insulated situations may prevent them from having access to the many authorities which have been consulted in arranging the materials for this work."—*Phil. Med. and Phys. Journal.*

MANUAL OF MATERIA MEDICA AND PHARMACY. By H. M. EDWARDS, M. D. and P. VAVASSEUR, M. D. comprising a concise Description of the Articles used in Medicine; their Physical and Chemical Properties; the Botanical Characters of the Medicinal Plants; the Formulæ for the Principal Officinal Preparations of the American, Parisian, Dublin, &c. Pharmacopœias; with Observations on the proper Mode of combining and administering Remedies. Translated from the French, with numerous Additions and Corrections, and adapted to the Practice of Medicine and to the Art of Pharmacy in the United States. By JOSEPH TOGNO, M. D. Member of the Philadelphia Medical Society, and E. DURAND, Member of the Philadelphia College of Pharmacy.

"It contains all the pharmaceutical information that the physician can desire, and in addition, a larger mass of information, in relation to the properties, &c. of the different articles and preparations employed in medicine, than any of the dispensatories, and we think will entirely supersede all these publications in the library of the *physician.*"—*Am. Journ. of the Medical Sciences.*

MEMOIR ON THE TREATMENT OF VENEREAL DISEASES WITHOUT MERCURY, employed at the Military Hospital of the Val-de-Grace. Translated from the French of H. M. J. Desruelles, M. D. &c. To which are added, Observations by G. J. Guthrie, Esq. and various documents, showing the results of this Mode of Treatment, in Great Britain, France, Germany, and America. 1 vol. 8vo.

MEDICINE, SURGERY, &c.

SURGICAL MEMOIRS of the CAMPAIGNS of RUSSIA, GERMANY, and FRANCE. Translated from the French of Baron Larrey. In 8vo. with plates.

A MANUAL of MEDICAL JURISPRUDENCE, compiled from the best Medical and Legal Works; comprising an account of—I. The Ethics of the Medical Profession; II. Charters and Laws relative to the Faculty; and III. All Medico-legal Questions, with the latest Decisions: being an Analysis of a course of Lectures on Forensic Medicine. By Michael Ryan, M. D. Member of the Royal College of Physicians in London, &c. First American edition, with additions, by R. Eglesfield Griffith, M. D. In 8vo.

"There is not a fact of importance or value connected with the science of which it treats, that is not to be found in its pages. The style is unambitious but clear and strong, and such as becomes a philosophic theme."—*Monthly Review.*

"It is invaluable to Medical Practitioners, and may be consulted safely by the Legal Profession."—*Weekly Dispatch.*

DIRECTIONS for MAKING ANATOMICAL PREPARATIONS, formed on the basis of Pole, Marjolin, and Breschet, and including the new method of Mr. Swan: by Usher Parsons, M. D. Professor of Anatomy and Surgery. In 1 vol. 8vo. with plates.

"It is compiled and prepared with judgment, and is the best and most economical companion the student can possess to aid him in the pursuit of this delightful department of his labors."—*Boston Med. & Surg. Journal, Sept. 27, 1831.*

"This is unquestionably one of the most useful works on the preparation of Anatomical Specimens ever published. It should be in the hands of every lover of Anatomy; and as attention now is more directed to the formation of museums, it will be found a very valuable book. Nothing is omitted that is important, and many new formulæ are introduced, derived from the author's experience, and from rare books, which he has had the industry to collect."—*N. Y. Medical Journal, August, 1831.*

A PRACTICAL GUIDE to OPERATIONS on the TEETH, by James Snell, Dentist. In 8vo. with plates.

PRINCIPLES of PHYSIOLOGICAL MEDICINE, including Physiology, Pathology, and Therapeutics, in the form of Propositions; and Commentaries on those relating to Pathology, by F. J. V. Broussais; translated by Isaac Hays, M. D. and R. E. Griffith, M. D. In 8vo.

ELEMENTS of PHYSIOLOGY, by Robley Dunglison, M. D. In 2 vols. 8vo. with numerous illustrations.

PRINCIPLES of SURGERY, by John Syme, Professor of Surgery in the University of Edinburgh. In 8vo.

PRACTICAL REMARKS on the NATURE and TREATMENT of FRACTURES of the TRUNK and EXTREMITIES; by Joseph Amesbury, Surgeon. In 8vo. with plates and wood-cuts.

PHYSIOLOGICAL MEDICINE

HISTORY OF CHRONIC PHLEGMASIÆ, OR INFLAM-MATIONS, founded on Clinical Experience and Pathological Anatomy, exhibiting a View of the different Varieties and Complications of these Diseases, with their various Methods of Treatment. By F. J. V. Broussais, M. D. Translated from the French of the fourth edition, by Isaac Hays, M. D. and R. Eglesfeld Griffith, M. D. Members of the American Philosophical Society, of the Academy of Natural Science, Honorary Members of the Philadelphia Medical Society, &c. &c. In 2 vols. 8vo.

EXAMINATION OF MEDICAL DOCTRINES AND SYS-TEMS OF NOSOLOGY, preceded by Propositions contain-ing the Substance of Physiological Medicine, by J. F. V Broussais, Officer of the Royal Order of the Legion of Hon-or; Chief Physician and First Professor in the Military Hos-pital for Instruction at Paris, &c. Third edition. Translated from the French, by Isaac Hays, M. D. and R. E. Grif-fith, M. D. In 2 vols. 8vo. *In the press.*

A TREATISE ON PHYSIOLOGY, Applied to Pathology. By F. J. V. Broussais, M. D. Translated from the French, by Drs. Bell and La Roche. 8vo. Third American edition, with additions.

"We cannot too strongly recommend the present work to the attention of our readers, and indeed of all those who wish to study physiology as it ought to be studied, in its application to the science of disease." "We may safely say that he has accomplished his task in a most masterly manner, and thus established his reputation as a most excellent physiologist and profound pathol-ogist."—*North American Med. and Surg. Journ. Jan.* 1827.

THE PRINCIPLES AND PRACTICE OF MEDICINE. By Samuel Jackson, M. D. Adjunct Professor of Medicine in the University of Pennsylvania. 8vo.

THE PRACTICE OF MEDICINE, upon the Principles of the Physiological Doctrine. By J. G. Coster, M. D. Trans-lated from the French.

An EPITOME of the PHYSIOLOGY, GENERAL ANA-TOMY, and PATHOLOGY of BICHAT. By Thomas Henderson, M. D. Professor of the Theory and Practice of Medicine in Columbia College, Washington City. 8vo.

"The Epitome of Dr. Henderson ought and must find a place in the library of every physician desirous of useful knowledge for himself, or of being instru-mental in imparting it to others, whose studies he is expected to superintend." —*N. A. Med. and Surg. Journ. No.* 15.

A TREATISE on FEVER, considered in the spirit of the new medical Doctrine. By J. B. Boisseau. Translated from the French.

MEDICINE, &c.

CHOLERA, as it recently appeared in the towns of Newcastle and Gateshead, including cases illustrative of its Physiology and Pathology, with a view to the establishment of sound principles of Practice. By T. M. GREENHOW, of Newcastle-upon-Tyne, Member of the Royal College of Surgeons in London, &c. &c. &c. In 1 vol. 8vo.

MANUAL OF GENERAL, DESCRIPTIVE, AND PATHOLOGICAL ANATOMY. By J. F. MECKEL, Professor of Anatomy at Halle, &c. &c. Translated from the French, with Notes, by A. SIDNEY DOANE, A. M. M. D. 3 vols. 8vo.

" It is among the most classical, learned, and authoritative treatises on Anatomy."—*American Journal of Med. Science.*

A PRACTICAL GUIDE TO OPERATIONS ON THE TEETH. By JAMES SNELL, Dentist. In 1 vol. 8vo. with Plates.

" Those of our readers who practise in the department of Surgery, on which Mr. Snell's essay treats, will find some useful instructions on the mode of extracting teeth."—*Med. Gazette.*
" This is an excellent practical work, and will be found generally useful."—*Athenæum.*
" This is the best practical manual for the dentist we have seen in the English language."—*Gaz. of Health.*

PRINCIPLES OF PHYSIOLOGICAL MEDICINE, including Physiology, Pathology, and Therapeutics, in the form of Propositions, and commentaries on those relating to Pathology, by F. J. V. BROUSSAIS, &c.; translated by ISAAC HAYS, M. D. and R. E. GRIFFITH, M. D. In 8vo.

" The present work will form an indispensable addition to the library of every physician. It is a very important and necessary companion to the Treatise on Physiology as applied to Pathology, by the same author."—*American Journal of Med. Science.*

PRINCIPLES OF SURGERY. By JOHN SYME, Professor of Surgery in the University of Edinburgh. In 8vo.

HUMAN PHYSIOLOGY, illustrated by numerous Engravings; by ROBLEY DUNGLISON, M. D., Professor of Physiology, Pathology, &c. in the University of Virginia, Member of the American Philosophical Society, &c. 2 vols. 8vo.

It is the most complete and satisfactory system of Physiology in the English language. It will add to the already high reputation of the author."—*American Journal of Med. Science.*

A TREATISE ON THE DISEASES OF THE EYE. By WILLIAM LAWRENCE, M. D. 1 vol. 8vo. *In the press.*

" It is almost unnecessary to say, that it contains marks of vast erudition and exact judgment, and that experience has dictated the principles that are comprised in them, experience drawn from a hospital devoted solely to the treatment of diseases of the Eye."—*Billard.*

A TREATISE ON DISEASES OF THE HEART AND GREAT VESSELS. By J. R. BERTIN. Edited by G. BOUILLAUD. Translated from the French. 8vo.

MEDICINE AND SURGERY.

A TREATISE ON FEVER. By SOUTHWOOD SMITH, M. D., Physician to the London Fever Hospital.

"No work has been more lauded by the Reviews than the Treatise on Fevers, by Southwood Smith. Dr. Johnson, the editor of the Medico-Chirurgical Review, says, 'It is the best we have ever perused on the subject of fever, and in our conscience, we believe it the best that ever flowed from the pen of physician in any age or in any country.'"—*Am. Med. Journ.*

AN ESSAY ON REMITTENT AND INTERMITTENT DISEASES, including generically Marsh Fever and Neuralgia—comprising under the former, various Anomalies, Obscurities, and Consequences, and under a new systematic View of the latter, treating of Tic Douloureux, Sciatica, Headache, Ophthalmia, Toothache, Palsy, and many other Modes and Consequences of this generic Disease; by JOHN MACCULLOCH, M. D., F. R. S. &c. &c.

"In rendering Dr. Macculloch's work more accessible to the profession, we are conscious that we are doing the state some service."—*Med. Chir. Review.*

"We most strongly recommend Dr. Macculloch's treatise to the attention of our medical brethren, as presenting a most valuable mass of information, on a most important subject."—*N. A. Med. and Surg. Journal.*

A PRACTICAL SYNOPSIS OF CUTANEOUS DISEASES, from the most celebrated Authors, and particularly from Documents afforded by the Clinical Lectures of Dr. Biett, Physician to the Hospital of St. Louis, Paris. By A. CAZENAVE, M. D and H. E. SCHEDEL, M. D.

"We can safely recommend this work to the attention of practitioners as containing much practical information, not only on the treatment, but also on the causes of cutaneous affections, as being in fact the best treatise on diseases of the skin that has ever appeared."—*American Journal of the Medical Sciences, No. 5.*

SURGICAL MEMOIRS OF THE RUSSIAN CAMPAIGN. Translated from the French of Baron LARREY.

LECTURES ON INFLAMMATION, exhibiting a view of the General Doctrines, Pathological and Practical, of Medical Surgery. By JOHN THOMPSON, M. D., F. R. S. E. Second American edition.

THE INSTITUTES AND PRACTICE OF SURGERY; being the Outlines of a Course of Lectures. By W. GIBSON, M. D. Professor of Surgery in the University of Pennsylvania. 3d edition, revised, corrected, and enlarged. In 2 vols. 8vo.

PRINCIPLES OF MILITARY SURGERY, comprising Observations on the Arrangements, Police, and Practice of Hospitals, and on the History, Treatment, and Anomalies of Variola and Syphilis; illustrated with cases and dissections. By JOHN HENNEN, M. D., F. R. S. E. Inspector of Military Hospitals—first American from the third London edition, with the Life of the Author, by his son, DR. JOHN HENNEN.

"The value of Dr. Hennen's work is too well appreciated to need any praise of ours. We were only required then, to bring the third edition before the notice of our readers; and having done this, we shall merely add, that the volume merits a place in every library, and that no military surgeon ought to be without it."—*Medical Gazette.*

ANATOMY.

DIRECTIONS FOR MAKING ANATOMICAL PREPARATIONS, formed on the basis of Pole, Marjolin and Breschet, and including the new method of Mr. Swan, by USHER PARSONS, M. D. Professor of Anatomy and Surgery. In 1 Vol. 8vo. with plates

A TREATISE ON PATHOLOGICAL ANATOMY. By WILLIAM E. HORNER, M. D. Adj. Prof. of Anatomy in the University of Pennsylvania.

"We can conscientiously commend it to the members of the profession, as a satisfactory, interesting, and instructive view of the subjects discussed, and as well adapted to aid them in forming a correct appreciation of the diseased conditions they are called on to relieve."—*American Journal of the Medical Science,* No. 9.

By the same Author.

A TREATISE ON SPECIAL AND GENERAL ANATOMY. Third edition, revised and corrected, in 2 Vols. 8vo.

LESSONS IN PRACTICAL ANATOMY, for the use of Dissectors. 2d edition, in 1 Vol. 8vo.

SYSTEM OF ANATOMY, for the use of Students of Medicine. By CASPAR WISTAR. Fifth edition, revised and corrected, by W. E. HORNER, Adjunct Professor of Anatomy in the University of Pennsylvania. In 2 Vols. 8vo.

ELEMENTS OF GENERAL ANATOMY, or a description of the Organs comprising the Human Body. By P. A. BECLARD, Professor of Anatomy to the Faculty of Medicine at Paris. Translated by J. TOGNO.

TREATISE ON SURGICAL ANATOMY. By ABRAHAM COLLES, Professor of Anatomy and Surgery, in the Royal College of Surgeons in Ireland, &c. Second American edition, with notes by J. P. HOPKINSON, Demonstrator of Anatomy in the University of Pennsylvania, &c. &c.

A TREATISE ON PATHOLOGICAL ANATOMY. By E. GEDDINGS, M. D. Professor of Anatomy in the Medical College of South Carolina. In 2 vols. 8vo. (In the press.)

ELEMENTS OF MYOLOGY. By E. GEDDINGS, M. D. illustrated by a series of beautiful Engravings of the Muscles of the Human Body, on a plan heretofore unknown in this country. *In the press.*

This work, in addition to an ample and accurate description of the general and special anatomy of the muscular system, will comprise illustrations of the subject from comparative anatomy and physiology, with an account of the irregularities, variations and anomalies, observed by the various ancient and modern anatomists, down to the present time.

CHEMISTRY.

THE CHEMISTRY OF THE ARTS, on the basis of Gray's Operative Chemist, being an Exhibition of the Arts and Manufactures dependent on Chemical Principles, with numerous Engravings, by ARTHUR L. PORTER, M. D. late Professor of Chemistry, &c. in the University of Vermont. In 8vo. With numerous Plates.

The popular and valuable English work of Mr. Gray, which forms the groundwork of the present volume, was published in London in 1829, and designed to exhibit a systematic and practical view of the numerous Arts and Manufactures which involve the application of Chemical Science. The author himself, a skilful, manufacturing, as well as an able, scientific chemist, enjoying the multiplied advantages afforded by the metropolis of the greatest manufacturing nation on earth, was eminently qualified for so arduous an undertaking, and the popularity of the work in England, as well as its intrinsic merits, attest the fidelity and success with which it has been executed. In the work now offered to the American public, the practical character of the Operative Chemist has been preserved, and much extended by the addition of a great variety of original matter, by numerous corrections of the original text, and the adaptation of the whole to the state and wants of the Arts and Manufactures of the United States. Among the most considerable additions will be found full and extended treatises on the Bleaching of Cotton and Linen, on the various branches of Calico Printing, on the Manufacture of the Chloride of Lime, or Bleaching Powder, and numerous Staple Articles used in the Arts of Dying, Calico Printing, and various other processes of Manufacture, such as the Salts of Tin, Lead, Manganese, and Antimony; the most recent Improvements on the Manufacture of the Muriatic, Nitric, and Sulphuric Acids, the Chromates of Potash, the latest information on the comparative Value of Different Varieties of Fuel, on the Construction of Stoves, Fire-Plates, and Stoving Rooms, on the Ventilation of Apartments, &c. &c. The leading object has been to improve and extend the *practical* character of the Operative Chemist, and to supply, as the publishers flatter themselves, a deficiency which is felt by every artist and manufacturer, whose processes involve the principles of chemical science, the want of a Systematic Work which should embody the most recent improvements in the chemical arts and manufactures, whether derived from the researches of scientific men, or the experiments and observations of the operative manufacturer and artisans themselves.

CHEMICAL MANIPULATION. Instruction to Students on the Methods of performing Experiments of Demonstration or Research, with accuracy and success. By MICHAEL FARADAY, F. R. S. First American, from the second London edition, with Additions by J. K. MITCHELL, M. D.

"After a very careful perusal of this work, we strenuously recommend it, as containing the most complete and excellent instructions for conducting chemical experiments. There are few persons, however great their experience, who may not gain information in many important particulars; and for ourselves, we beg most unequivocally to acknowledge that we have acquired many new and important hints on subjects of even every-day occurrence."—*Philosophical Mag.*

"A work hitherto exceedingly wanted in the laboratory, equally useful to the proficient and to the student, and eminently creditable to the industry and skill of the author, and to the school whence it emanates."—*Journal of Science and Arts.*